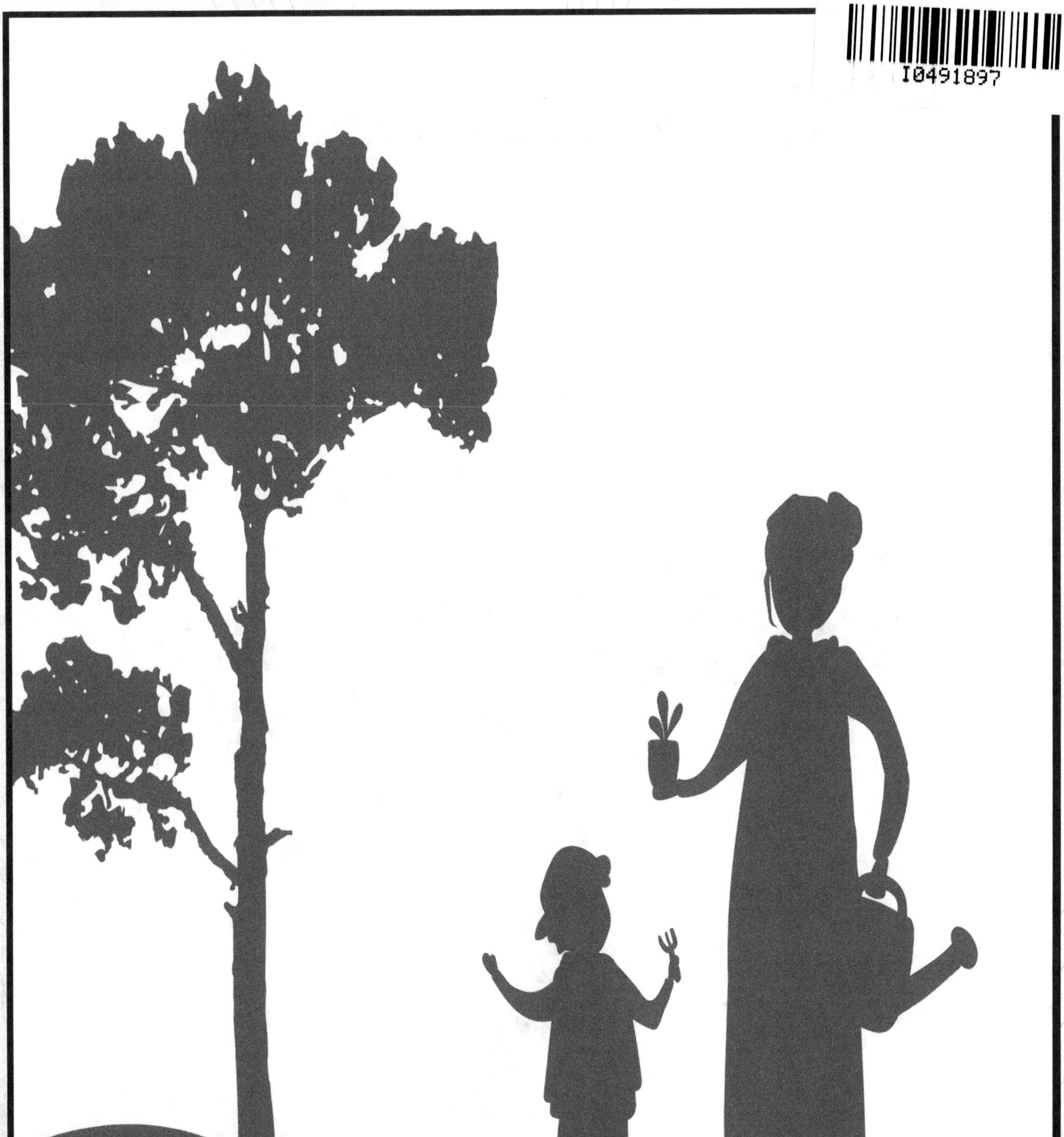

Copyright © 2021 · Alber Doncos · All rights reserved.

This book belongs to:

_____

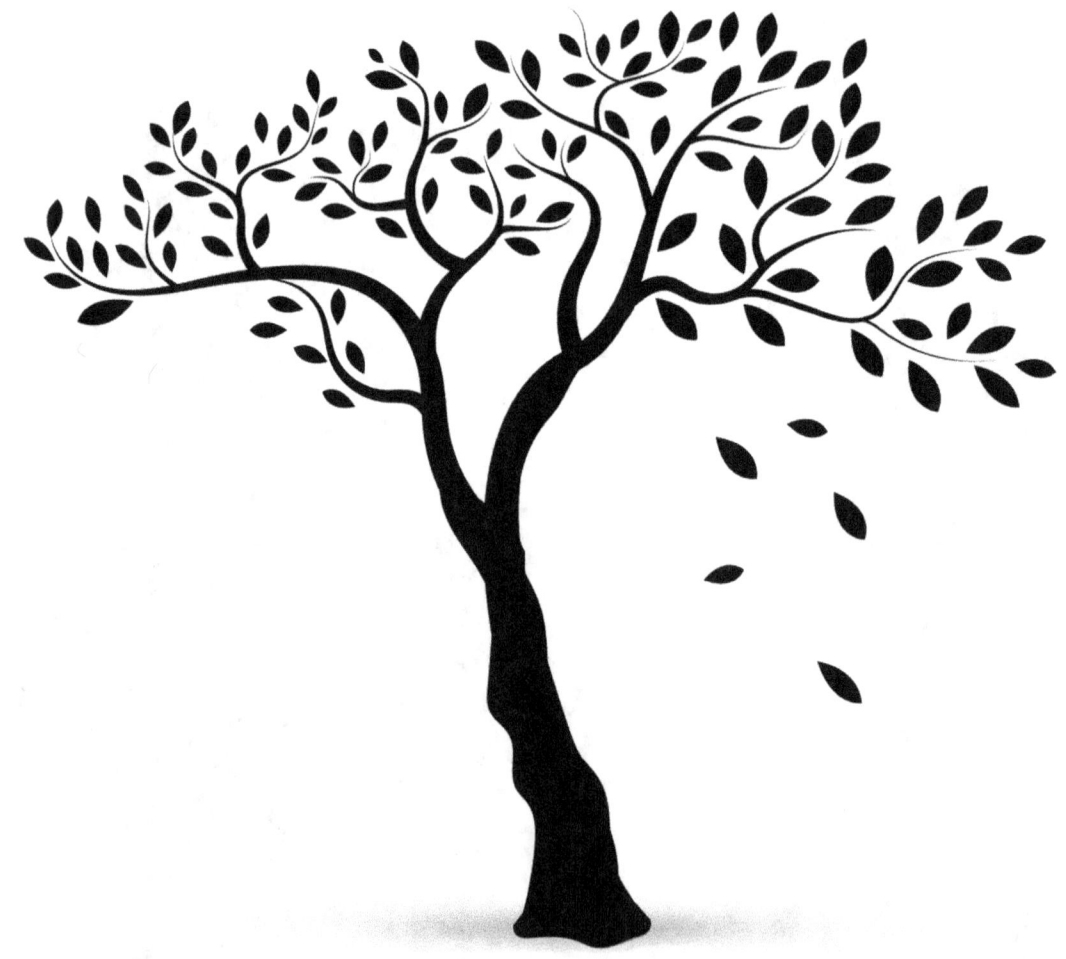

This book has been created and designed with the highest respect and
admiration for our elders, the people who have given us
life and from whom we have learned so much.
In moments like these we can give back to them in some ways,
at least a part of what they did for us...

Where were you born?

___

What are your parent's names?

___

Do you have any pets?

___

In what places have you lived?

___

Would you change something in your life?

___

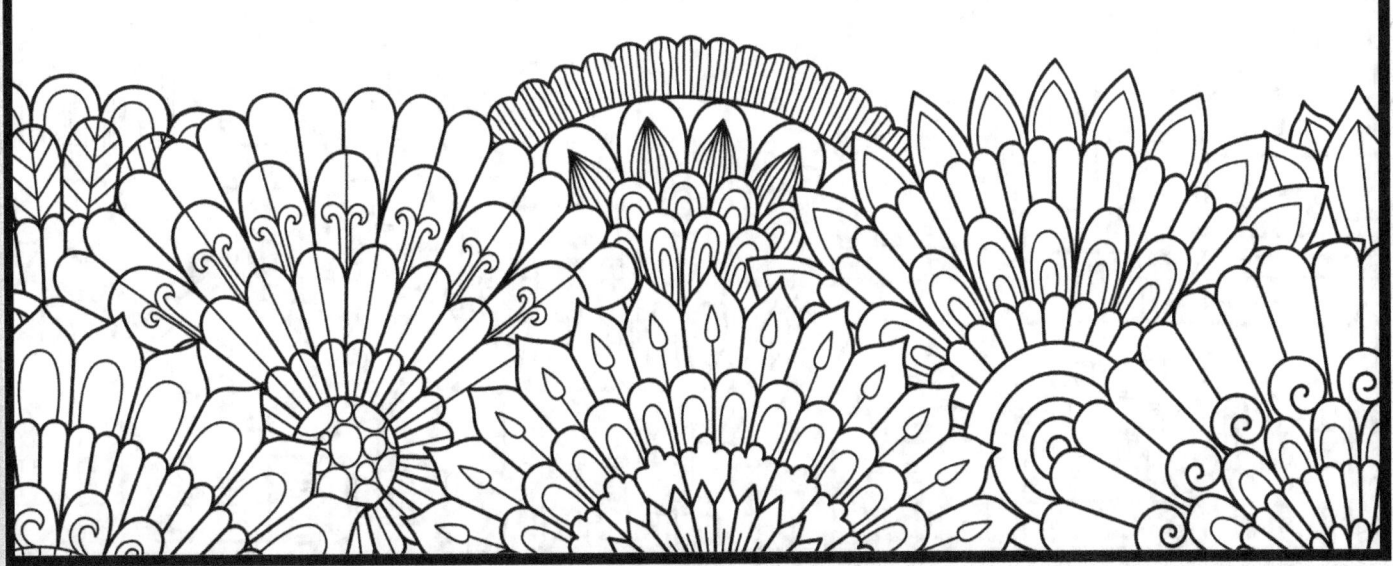

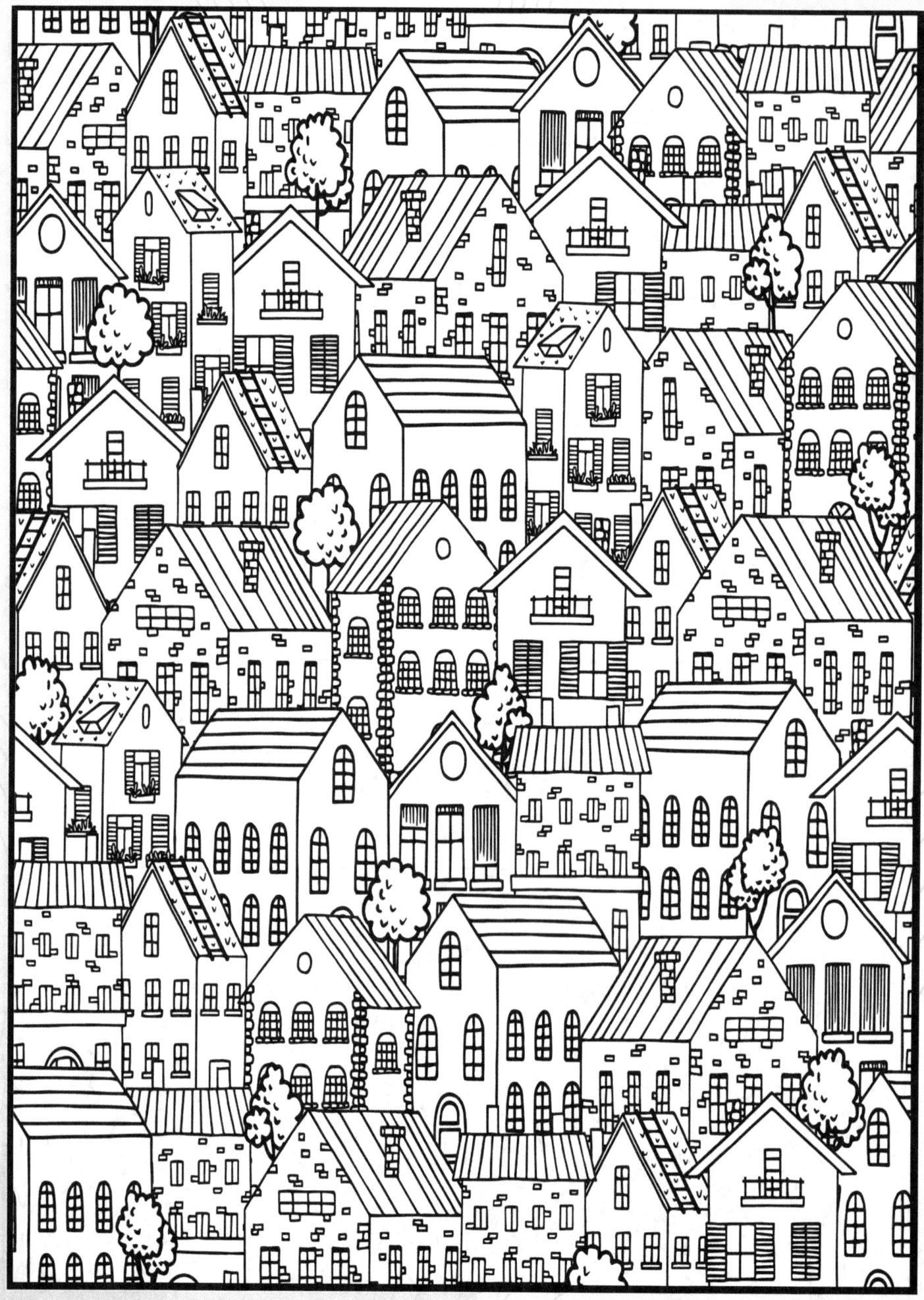

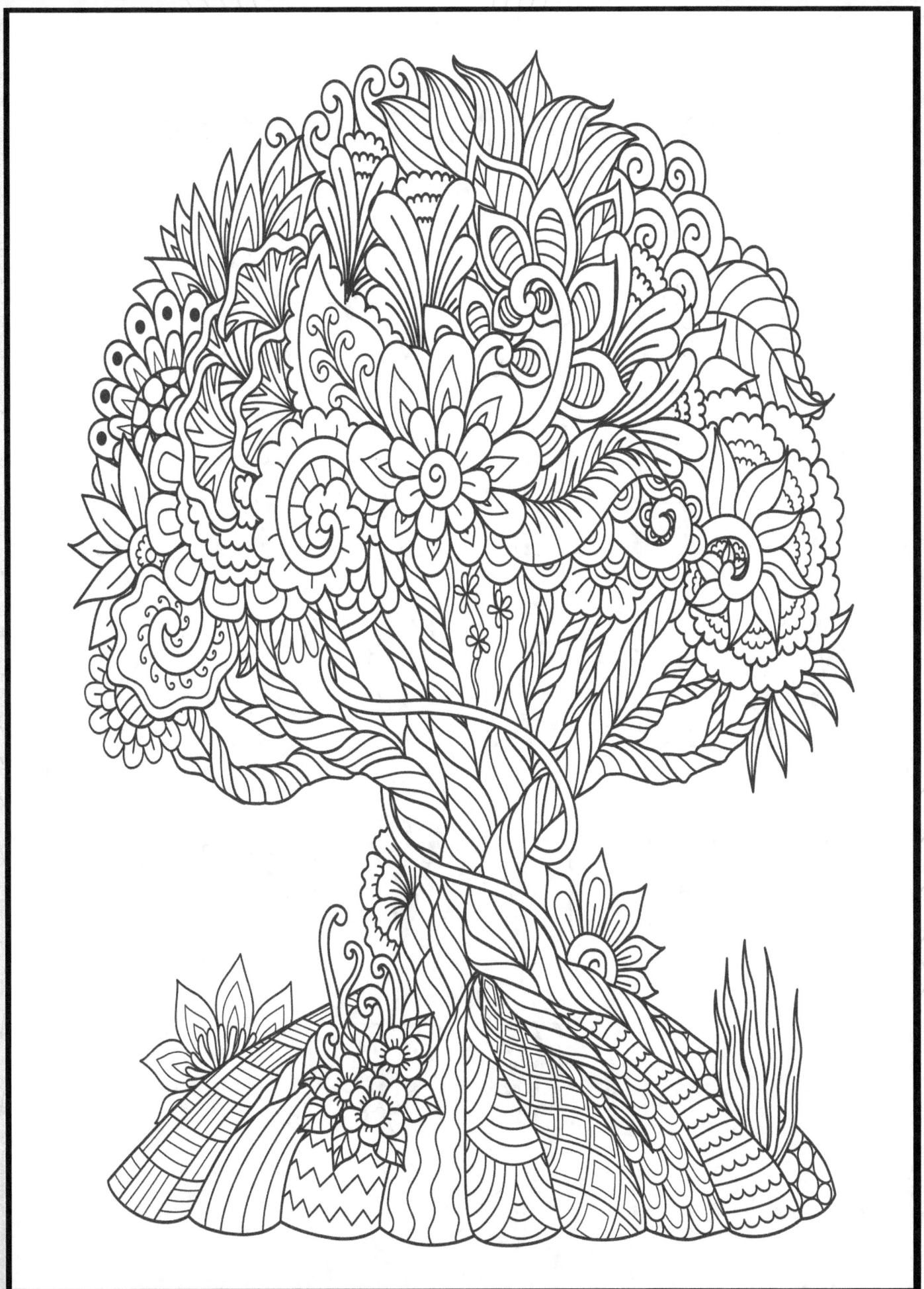

Do you remember the alphabet?

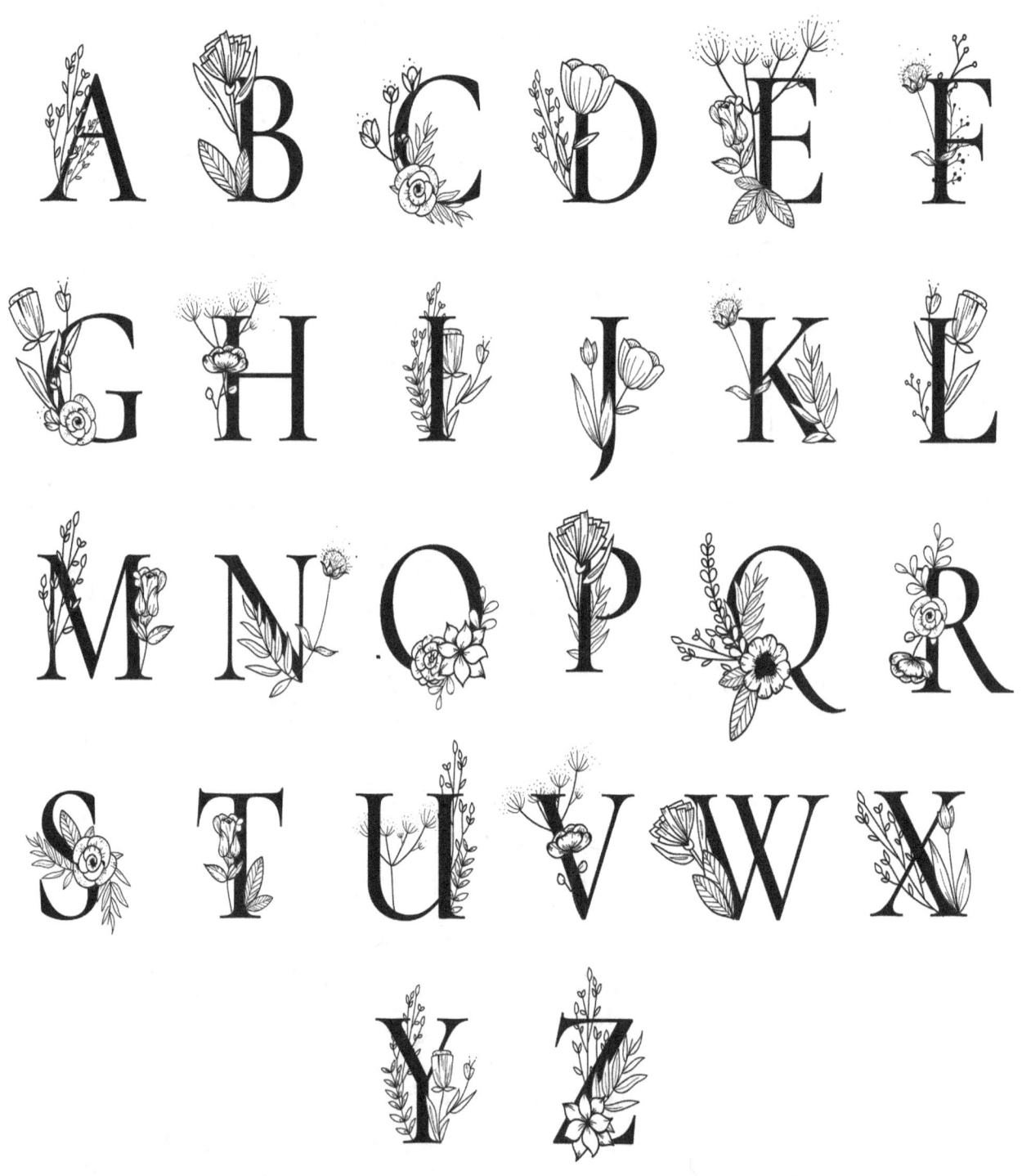

Write it here as many times as you can

_____

_____

_____

_____

_____

_____

_____

_____

_____

abcdefghi
jklmnopq
rstuvwxyz

Fill in your family tree

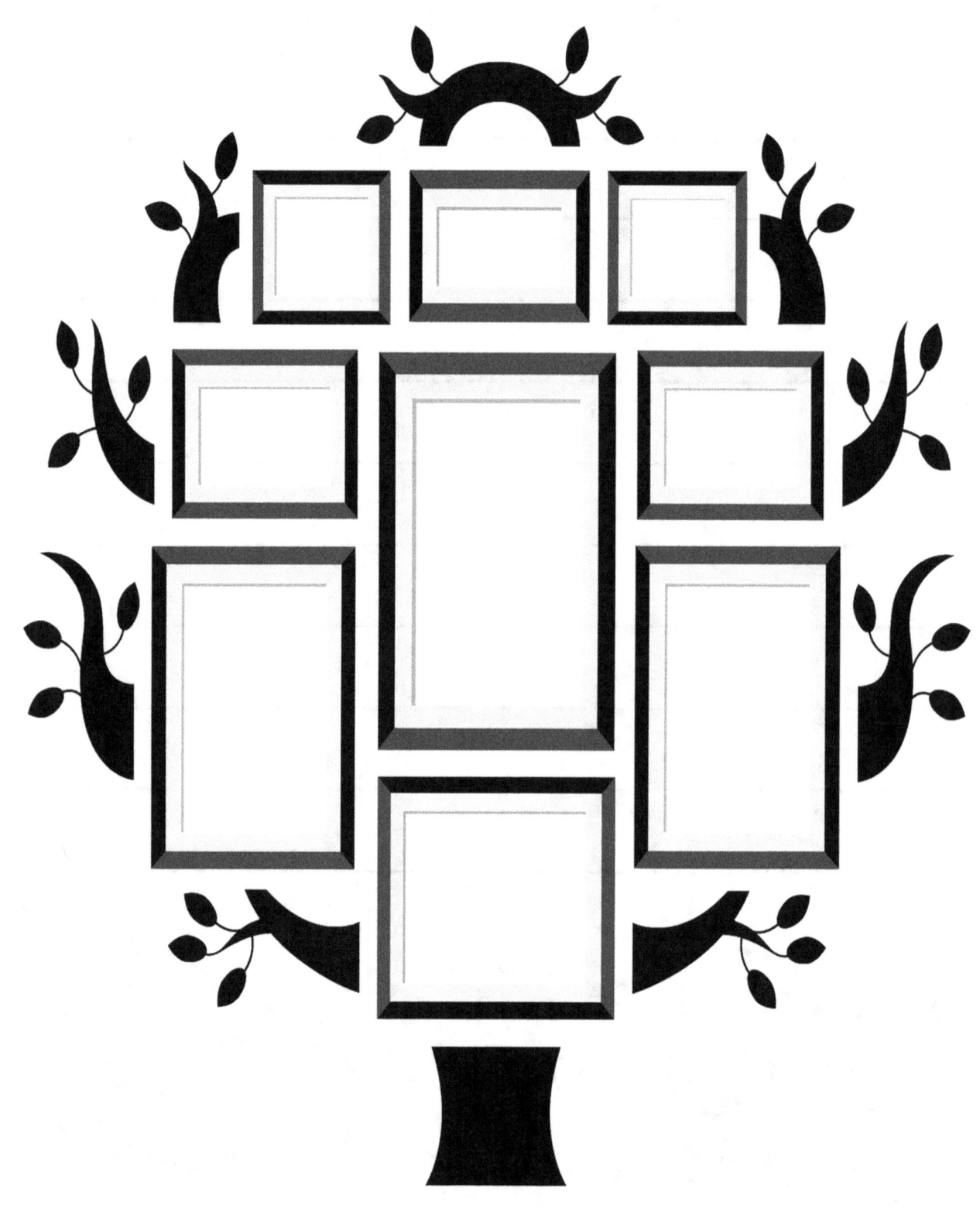

Paste a picture of your family here

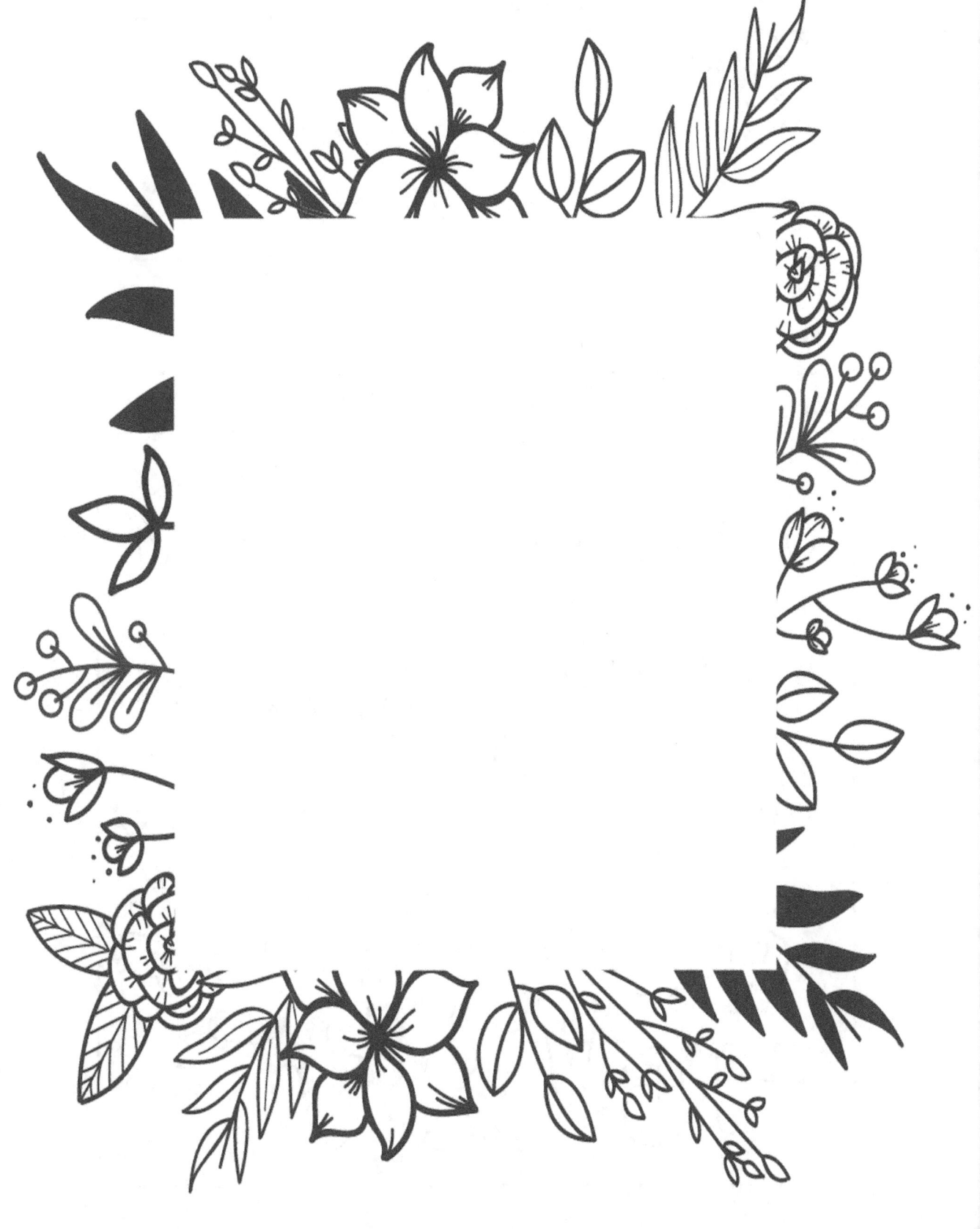

Trace

A A A A A A A A A A

a a a a a a a a a a a a a

Find and color A

A K a Z c D
O A K S A h
D M A e f a
a E a A a v
E G E k
H C y A d a

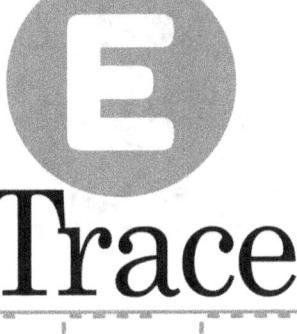

Trace

Find and color E

E H L e n f i ø A
B E c G i a E A
k a E E ε G f D
O S e · e E
e C J b d S E I F
G E i m k w e

Proverbs & Sayings

Barking dogs_____

_____than never

Better safe_____

_____ the wind to the shorn lamb

Every cloud has a _____

_____last, laughs best

Monkey see,_____

_____a bad name and hang it

A man is known by the_____

_____are grey in the dark

Proverbs & Sayings

Knowledge is no_____

_____enough to the wise

Easier said than done_____

_____ in time saves nine

Every law has its_____

_____a tooth for a tooth

A bird in the hand is worth _____

_____something new every day

Birds of a feather _____

_____cured must be endured

Make a circle to the elements that we can find in a kitchen

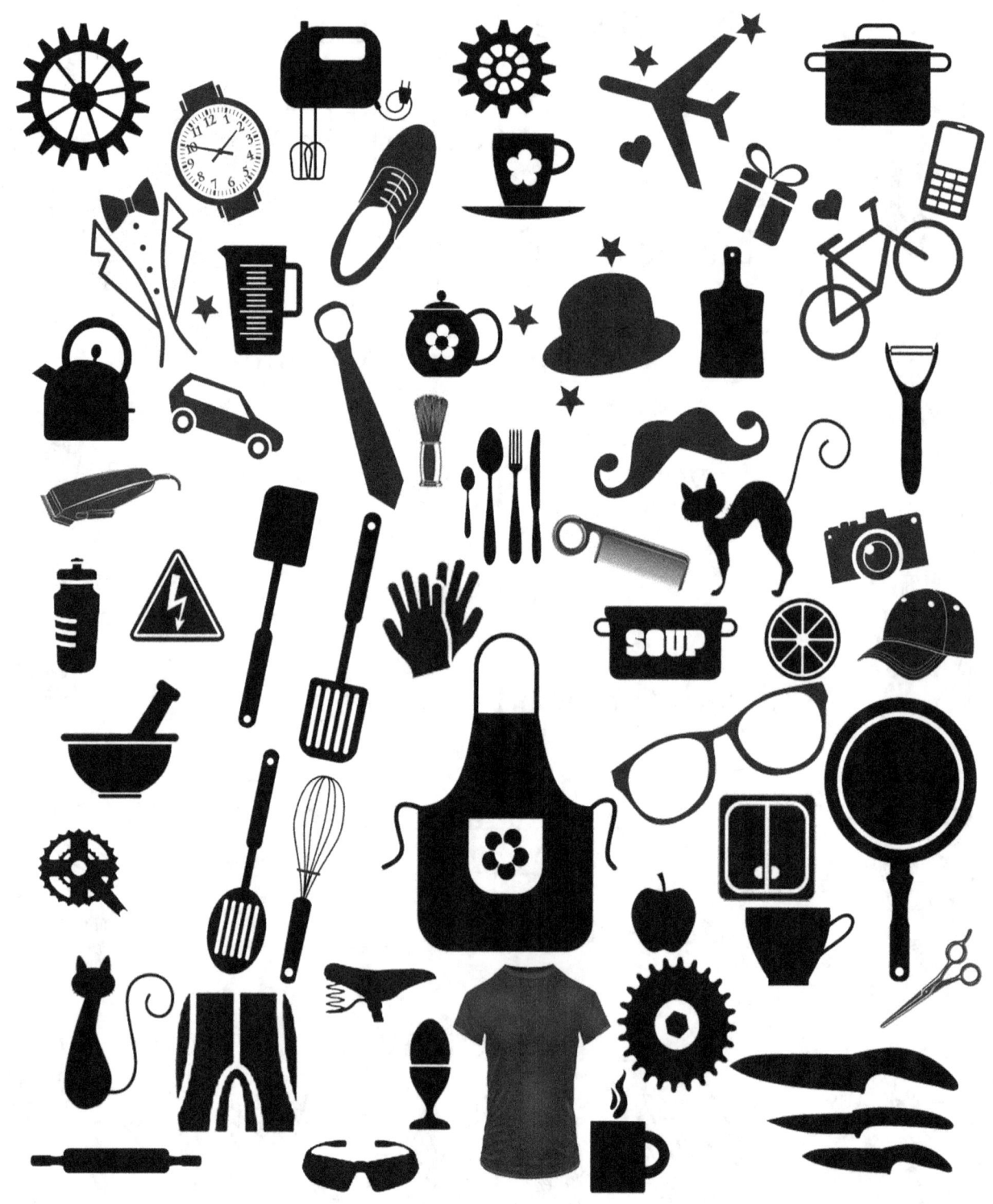

Write the name of each animal

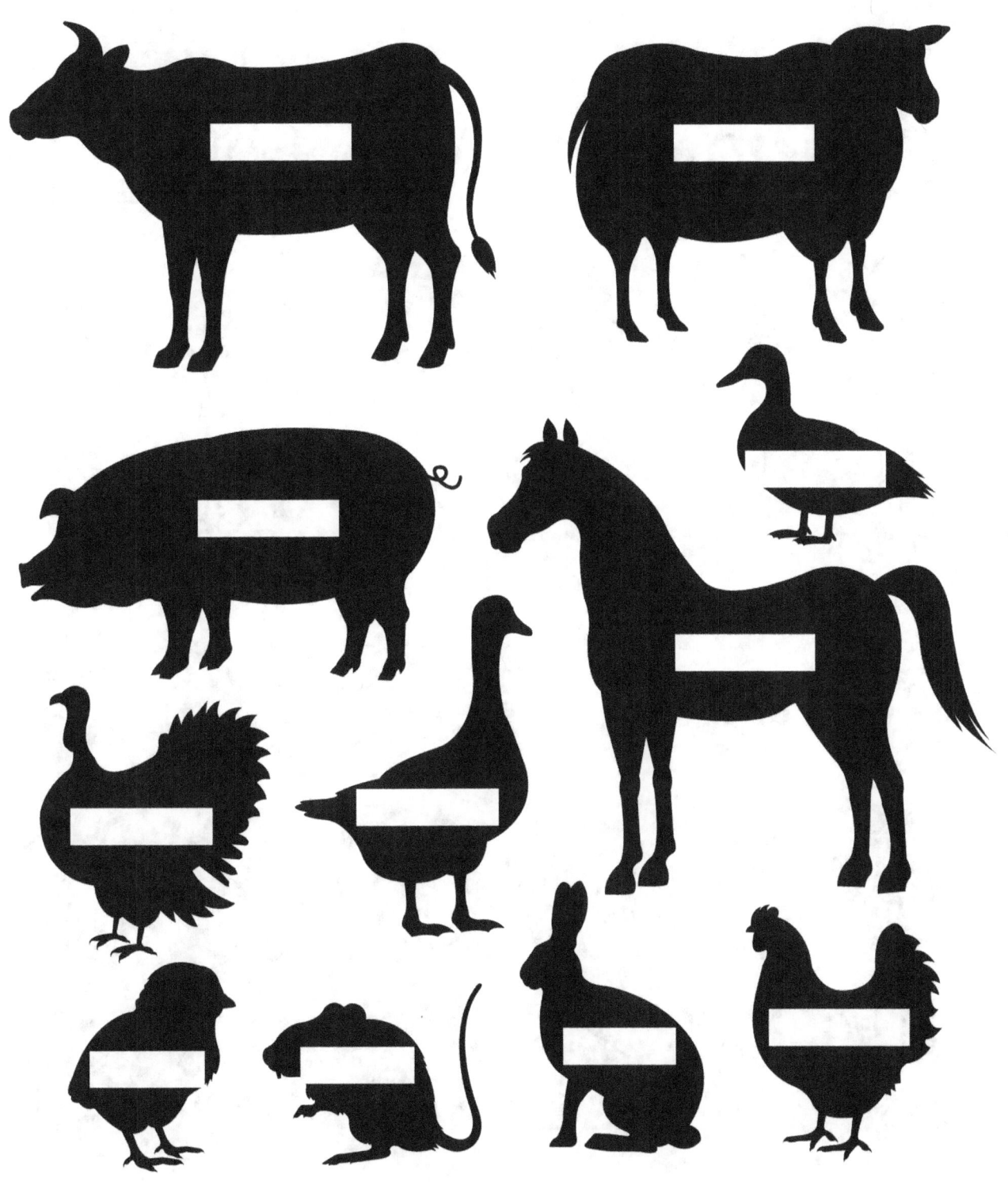

Find the pairs and match them

What is the different figure?

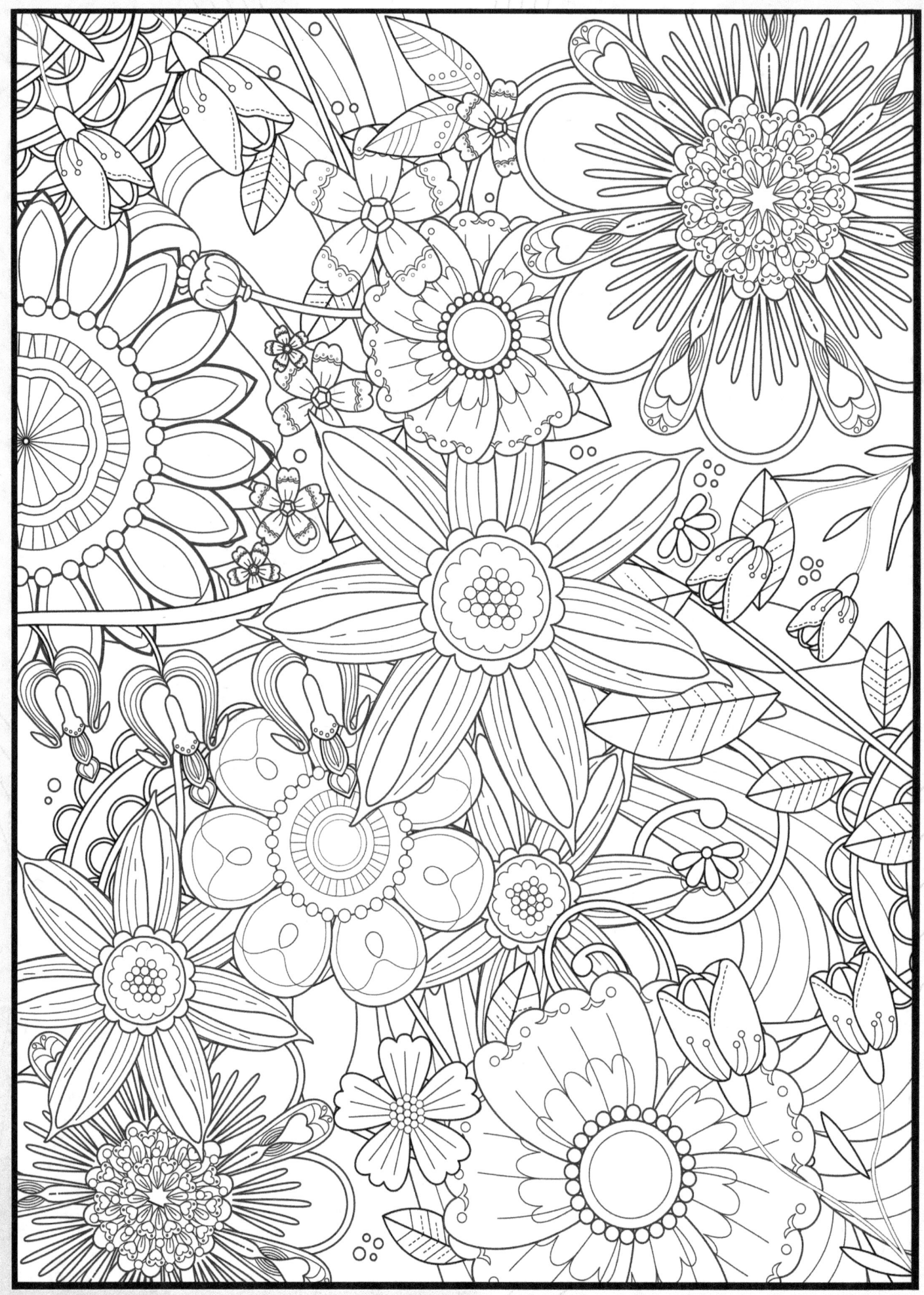

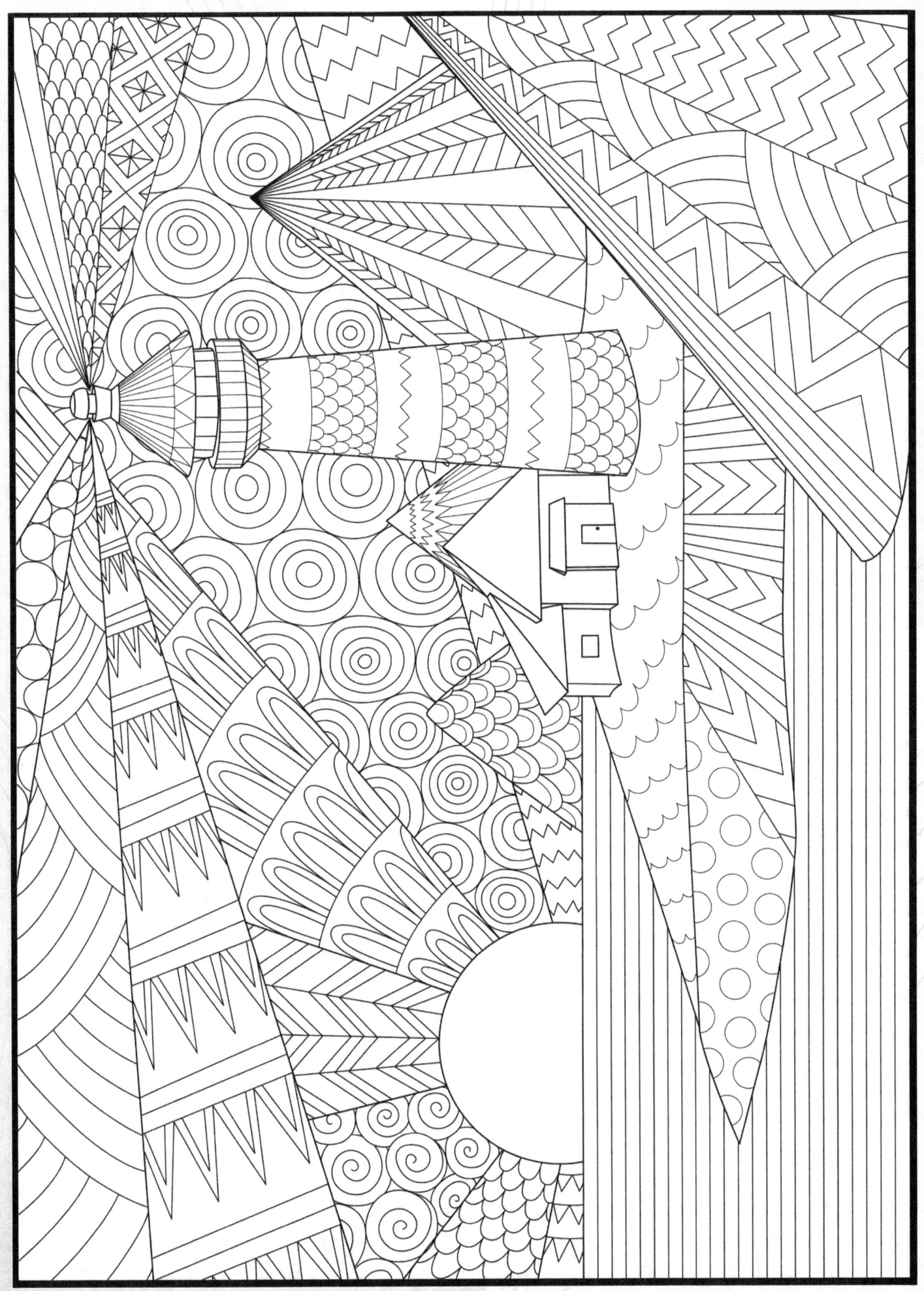

TRACE THE NUMBER

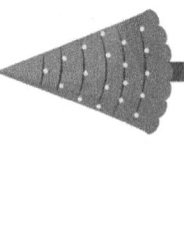

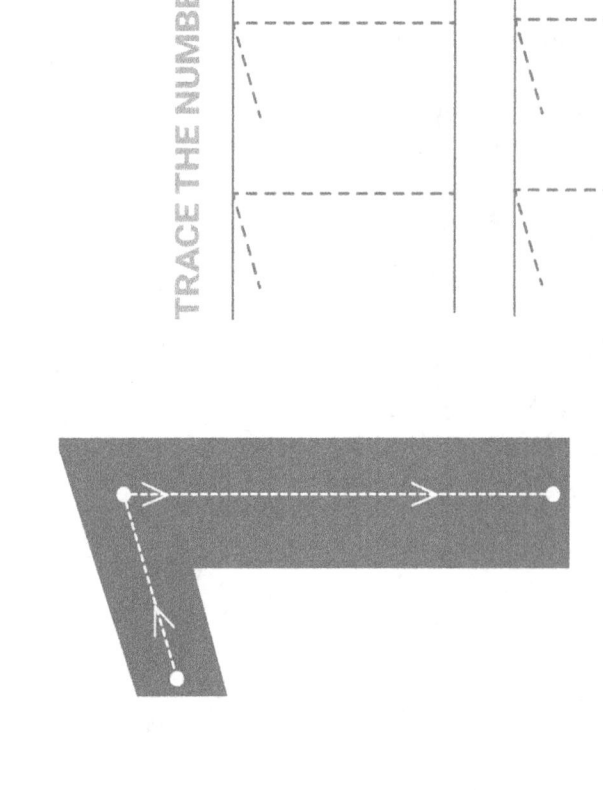

CLOLOR ONE CIRCLE

○ ○ ○ ○ ○
○ ○ ○ ○ ○

CIRCLE ALL THE NUMBER ONE

1 2 3 4 5

2 3 1 1 1

5 2 4 1 4 5

5

ONE

TRACE THE NUMBER

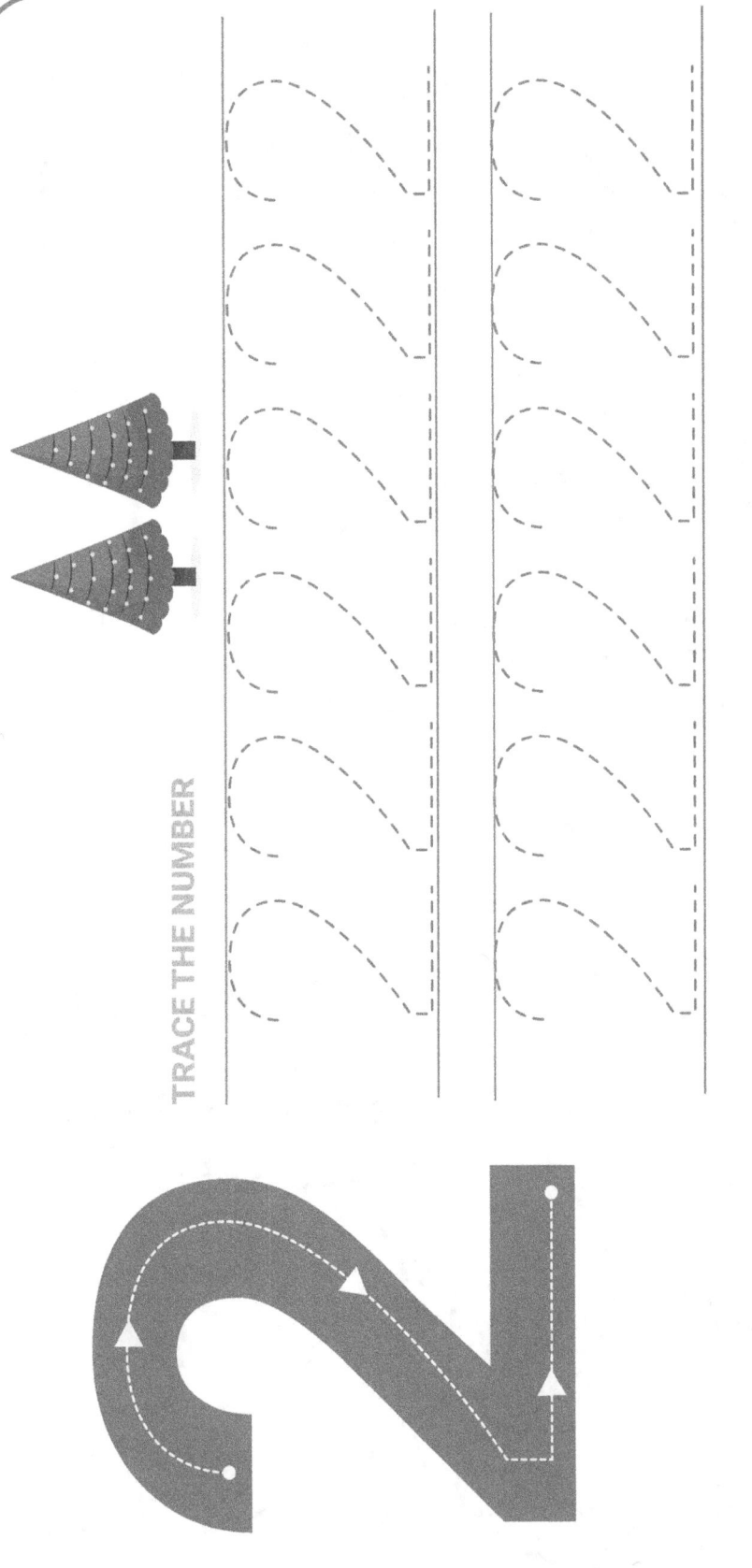

2

CIRCLE ALL THE NUMBER TWO

1 2 3 4 5
2 3 1 1 5
2 3 2 3 1
5 2 4 1 4
5 5 3

COLOR ONE CIRCLE

TWO

Find the 10 differences

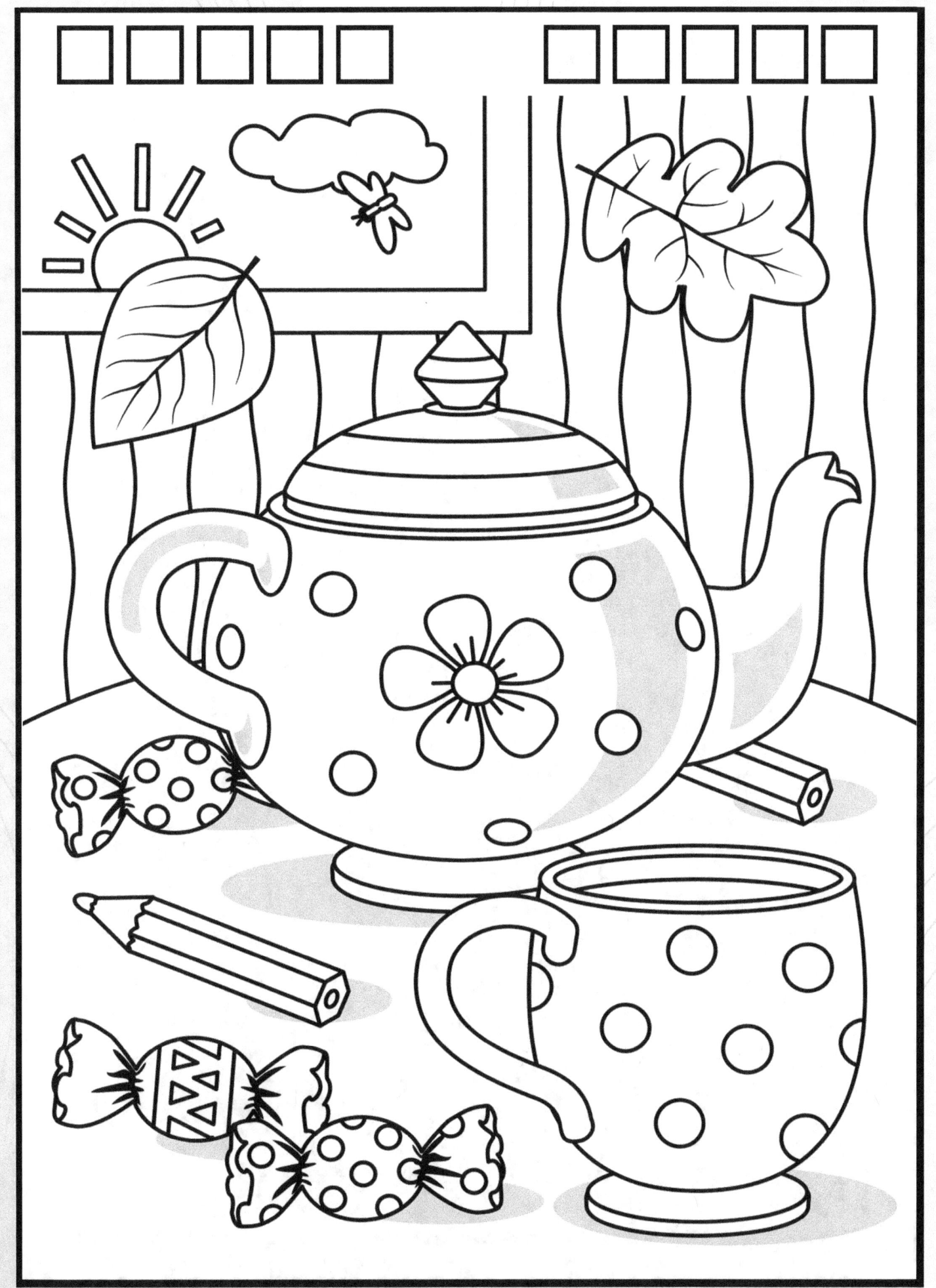

How many of each are there?

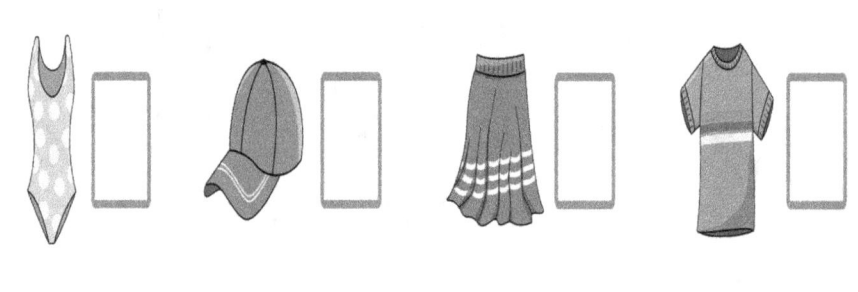

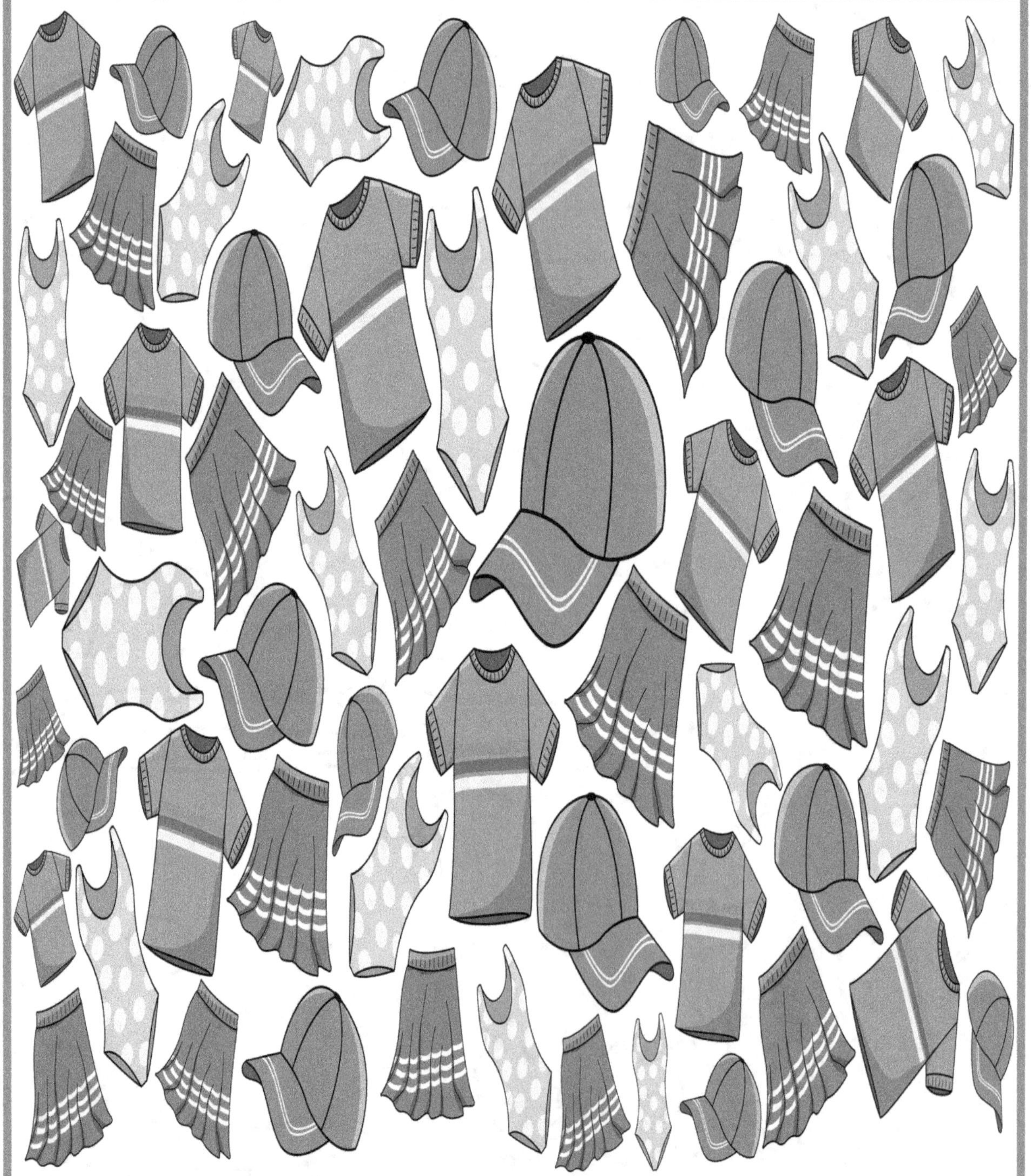

Write below each one the type of clock it is

Find the 2 cacti
that have the same shape

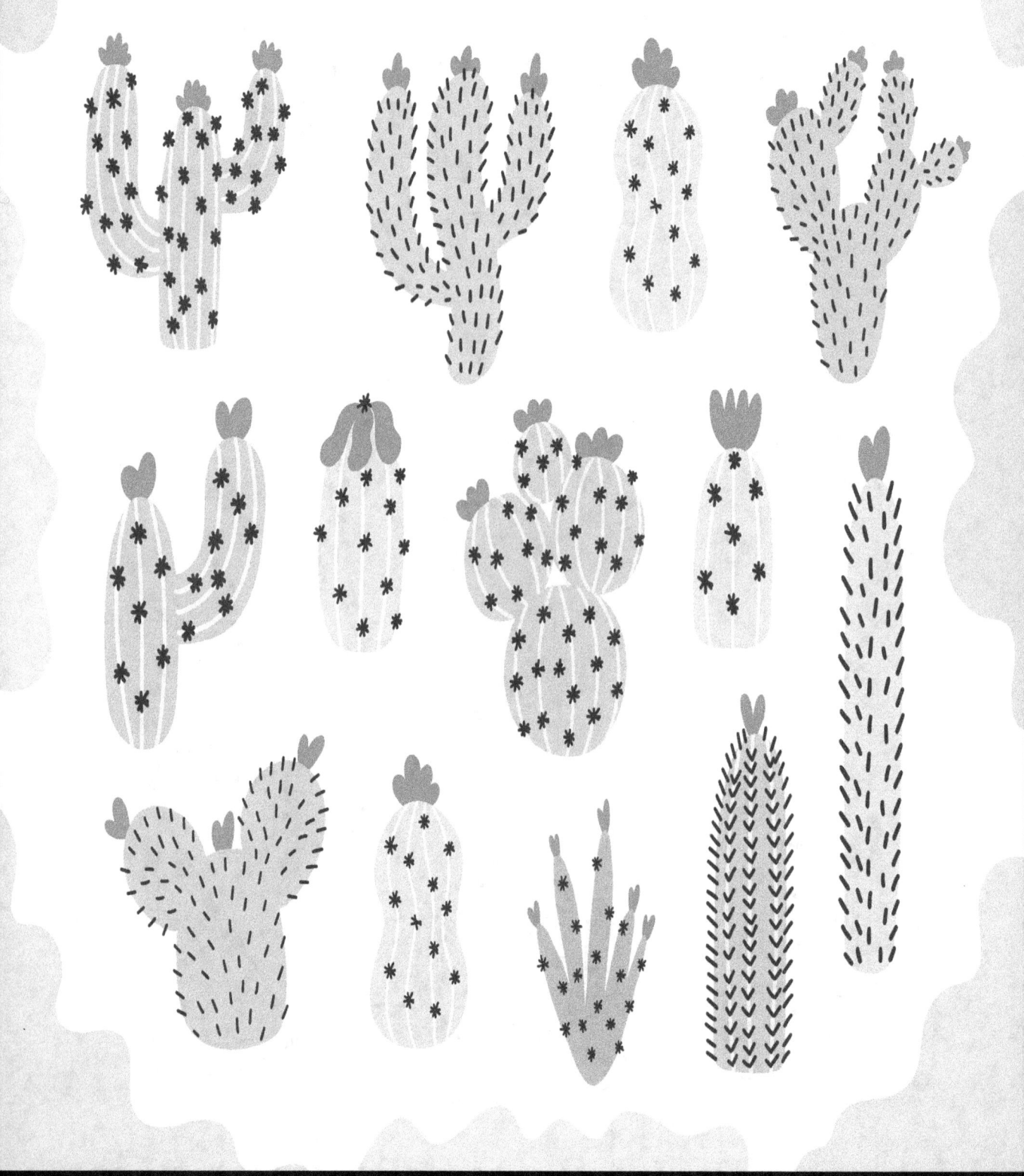

What is the best memory you have of your partner?

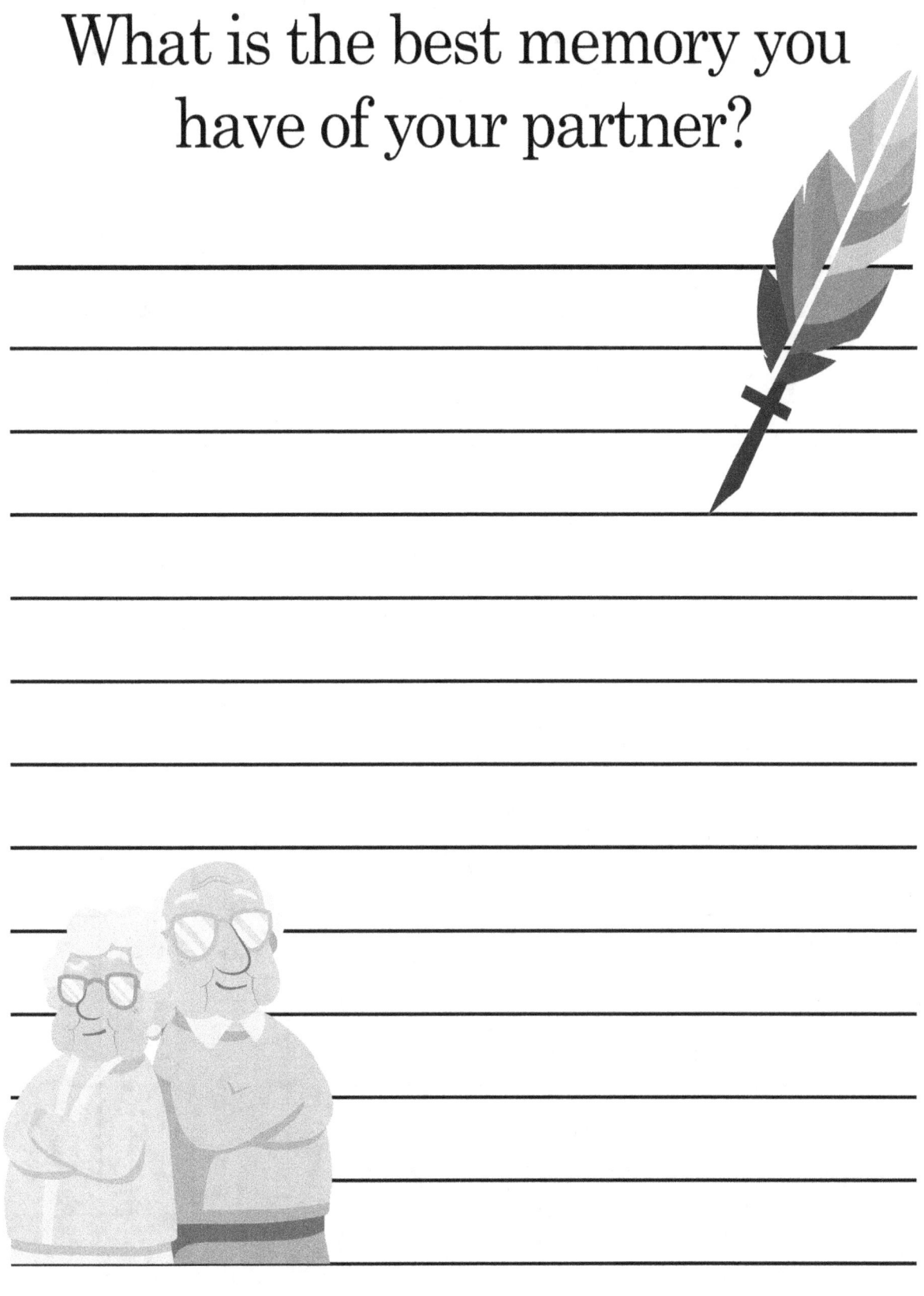

Can you help the cat find food?

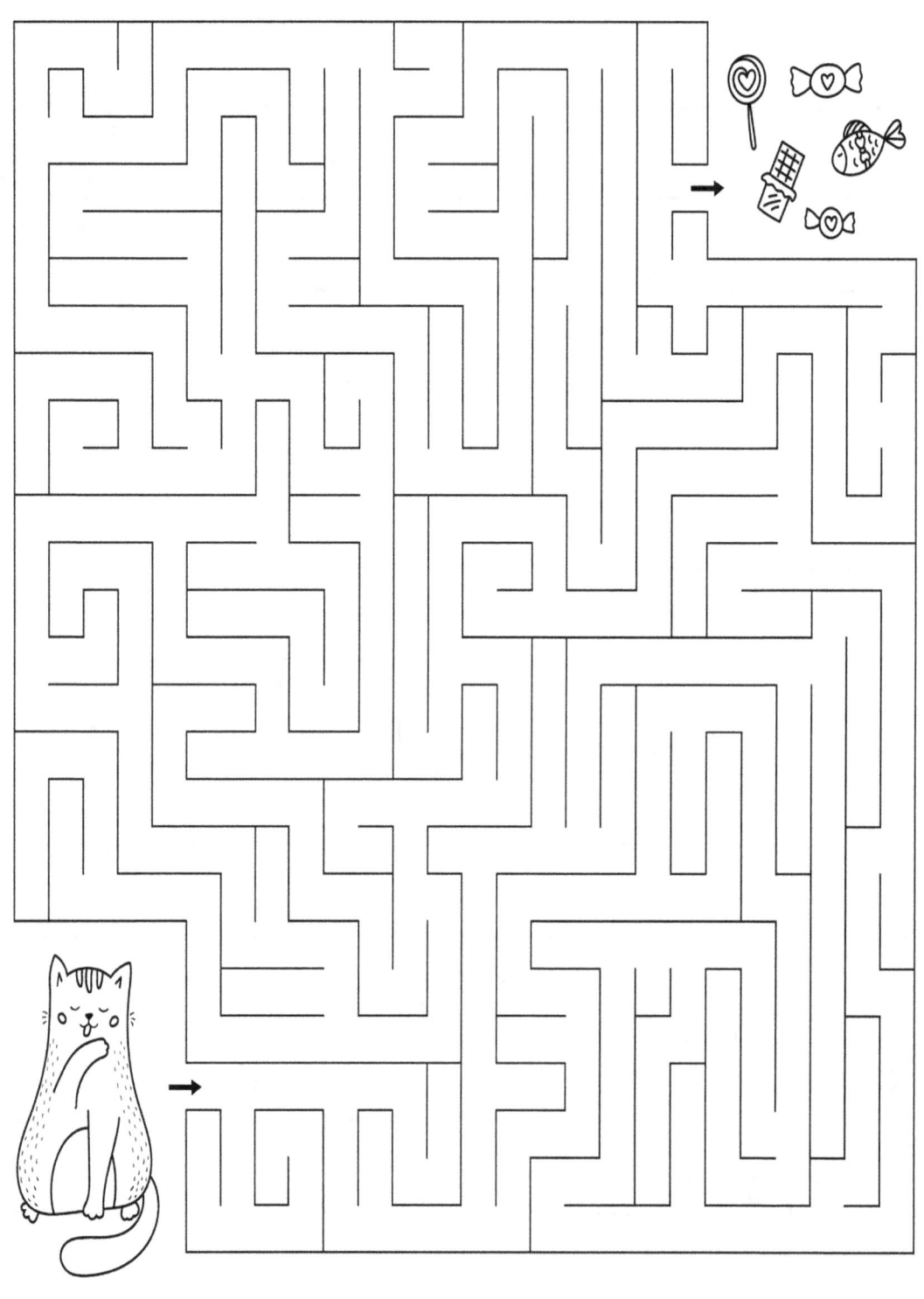

Count and match

6 + 7 ·	· 6
1 + 5 ·	· 17
5 + 6 ·	· 12
10 + 2 ·	· 13
7 + 10 ·	· 11

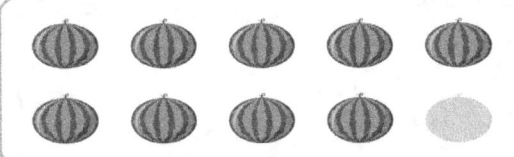

· ·	10
· ·	1
· ·	9
· ·	6

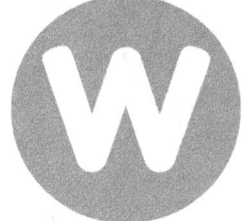

TRACE

Find and color W

A Y S t W Z W
W W J H M R
Y i m W K W
i W D R W O
C W G W M V
M L W W F W

TRACE

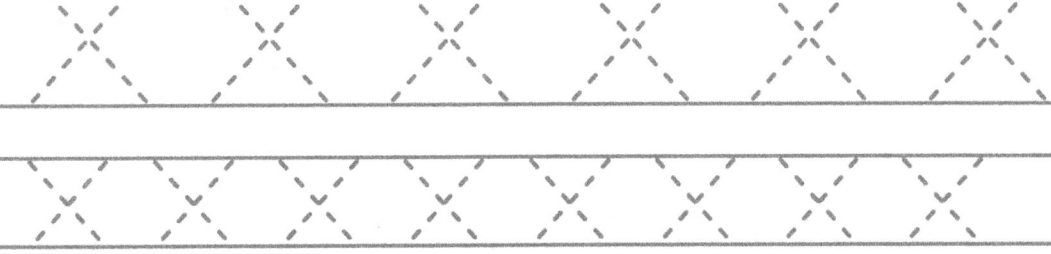

Find and color X:

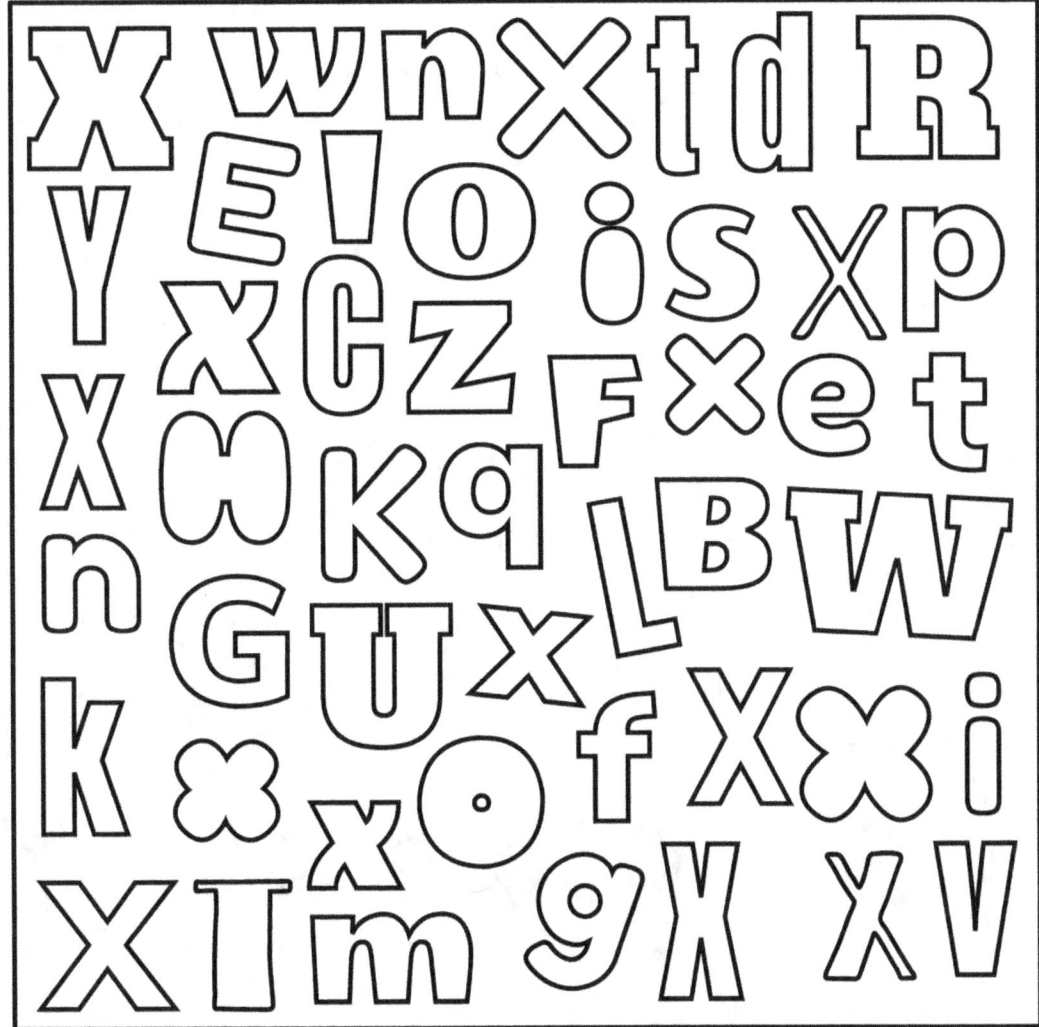

Mark each dotted line with a different color

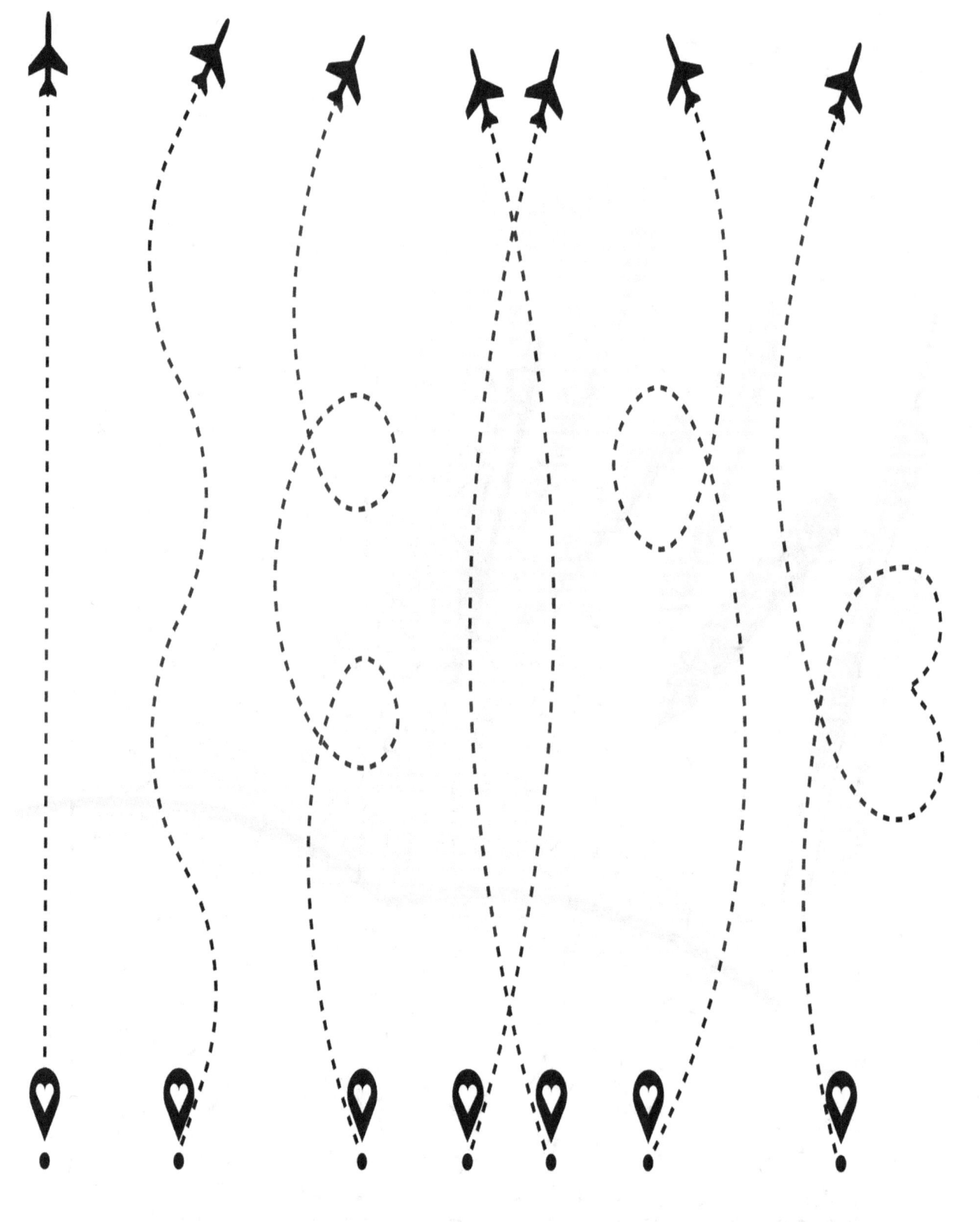

Write the result

$$1 \times 3 = \square$$

$$2 \times 2 = 6$$

$$6 \times \square = 0$$

$$4 \times \square = \square$$

$$\square \times 4 = 8$$

$$3 \times \square = 6$$

$$\square \times 2 = \square$$

$$\square \times 0 = \square$$

$$\square \times 1 = \square$$

$$\square \times 10 = \square$$

Vertical equations:
- $1 \times \square \times 6 = \square$
- $3 \times \square \times 3 = \square$
- $7 \times \square = 0$
- $2 \times \square = 4$
- $6 \times \square = 5$
- $2 \times \square = \square$ (with $\square$) $= \square$

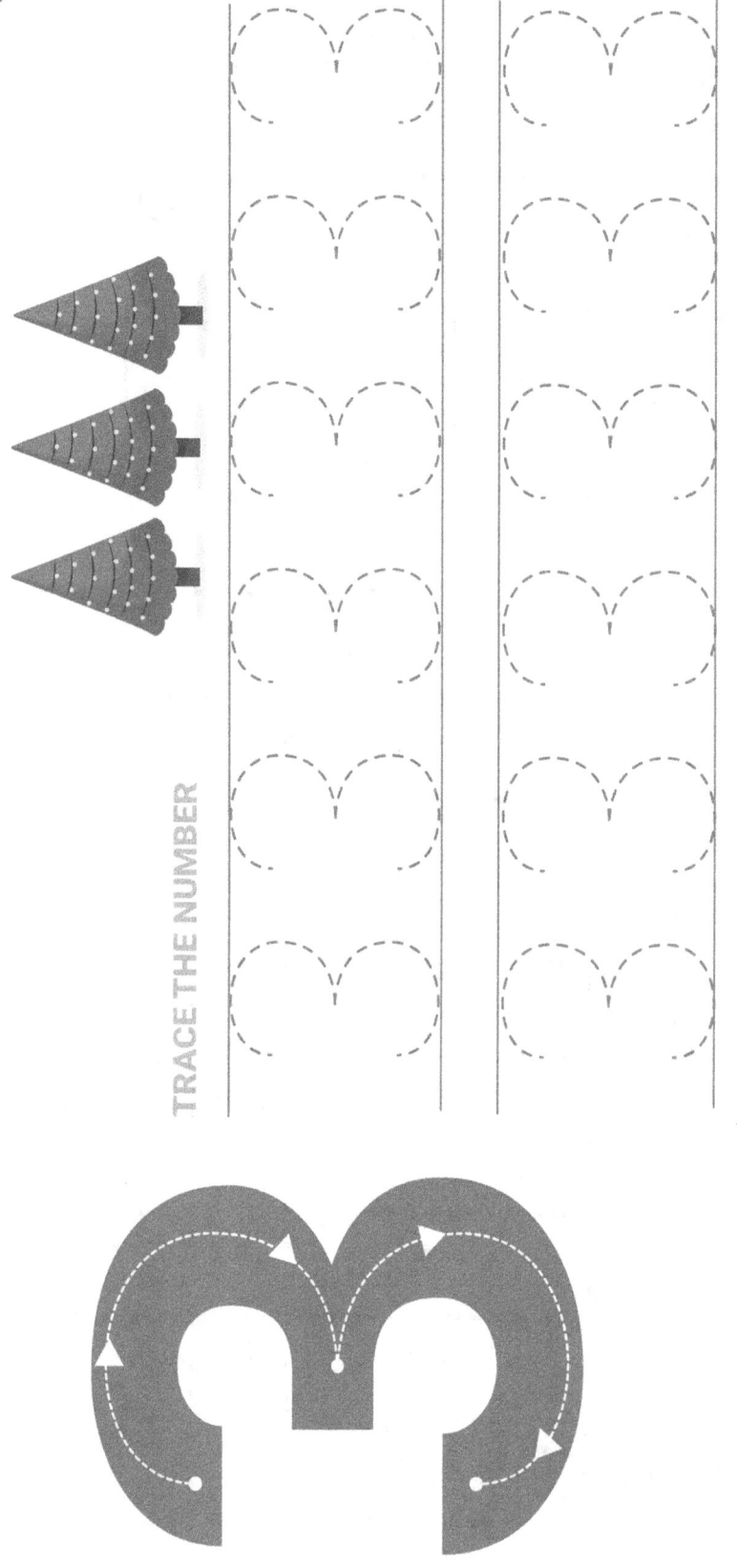

TRACE THE NUMBER

CIRCLE ALL THE NUMBER TREE

1	2	3	4	5
	2	3	1	1
	2	3	2	3	1
5	2	4	4	5
		5	1	3

CLOLOR ONE CIRCLE

THREE

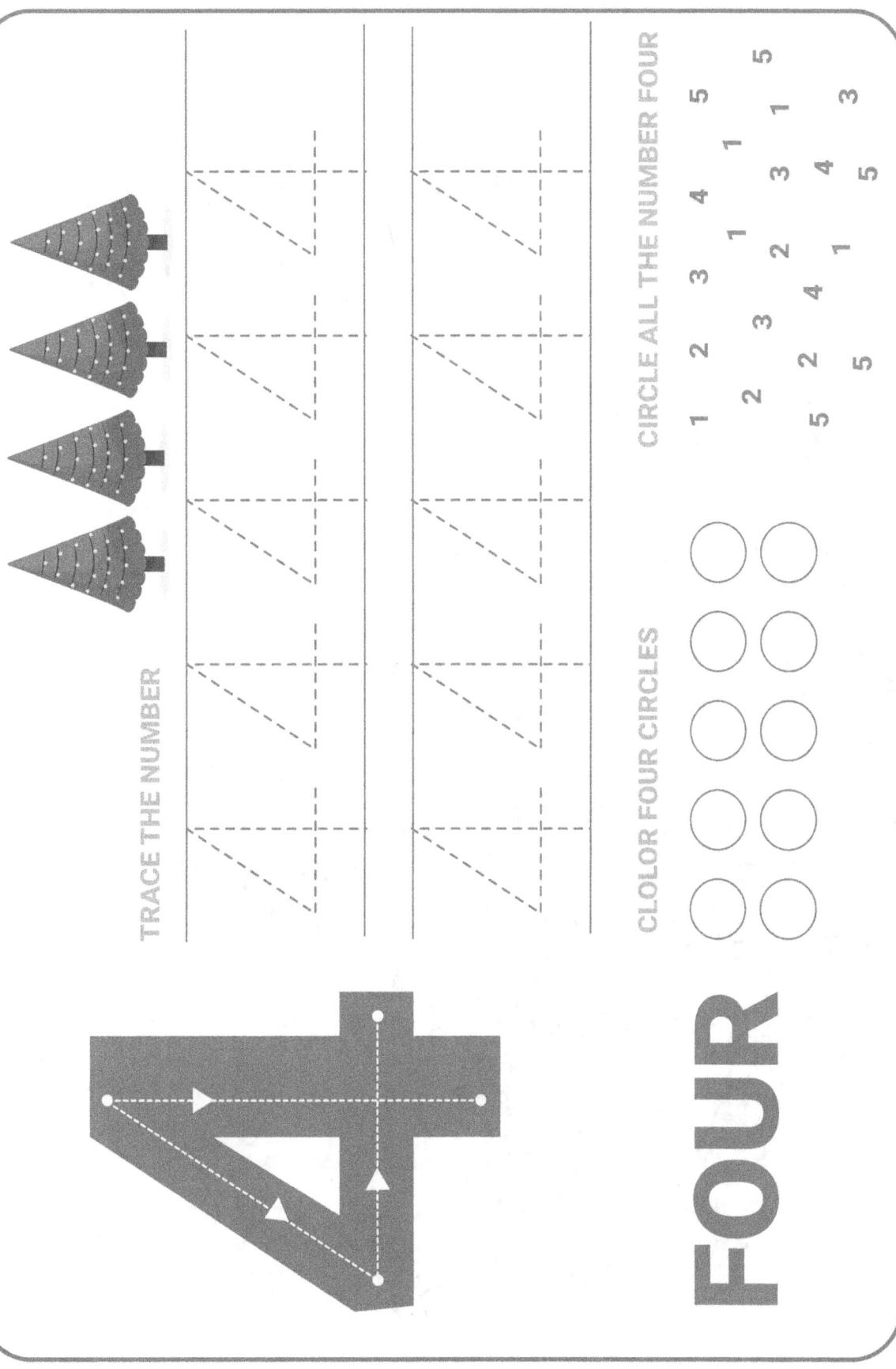

TRACE THE NUMBER

CLOLOR FOUR CIRCLES

CIRCLE ALL THE NUMBER FOUR

1 2 3 4 5
2 3 1 1 1
5 2 4 3 1
5 1 4 5
5 3

FOUR

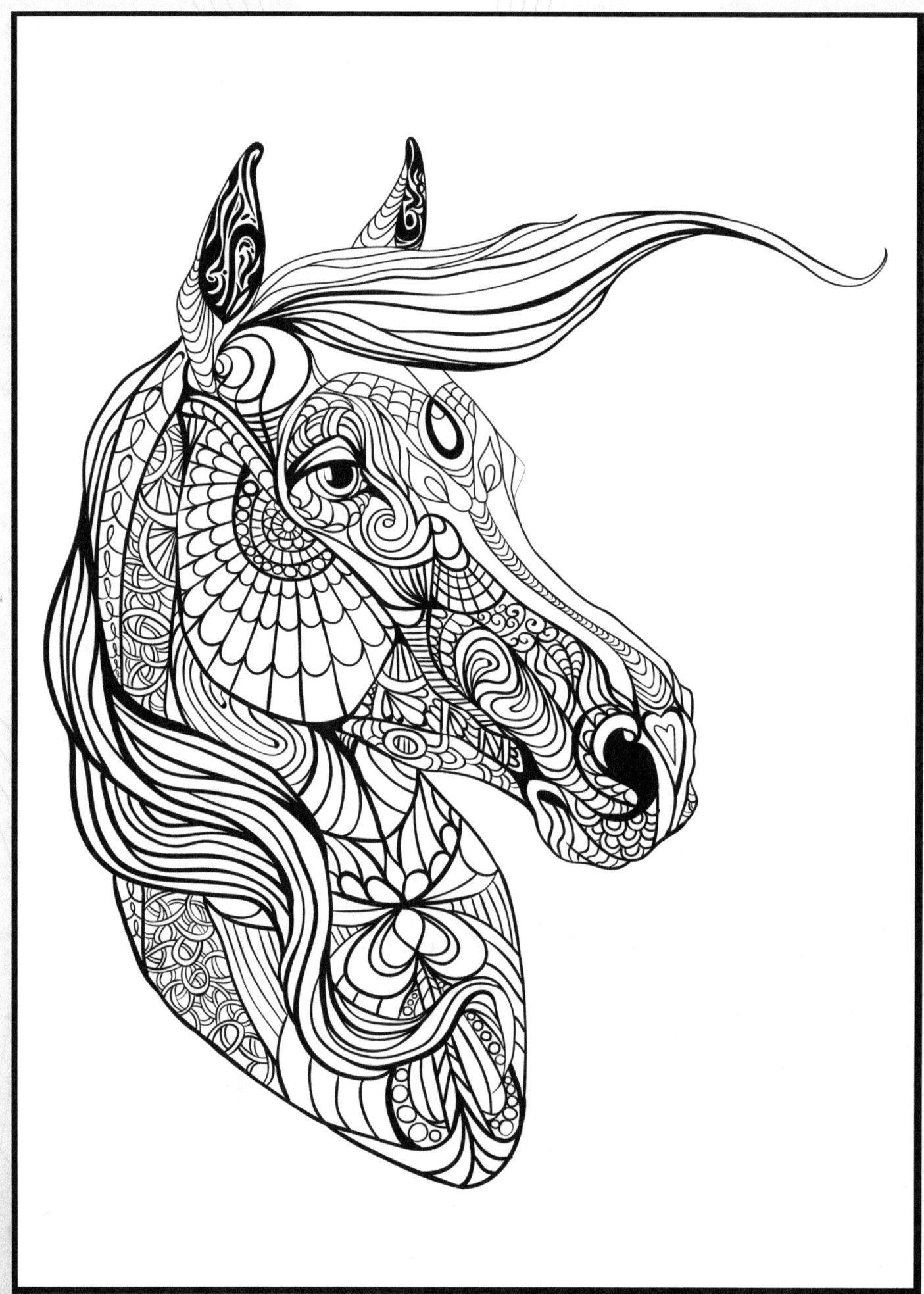

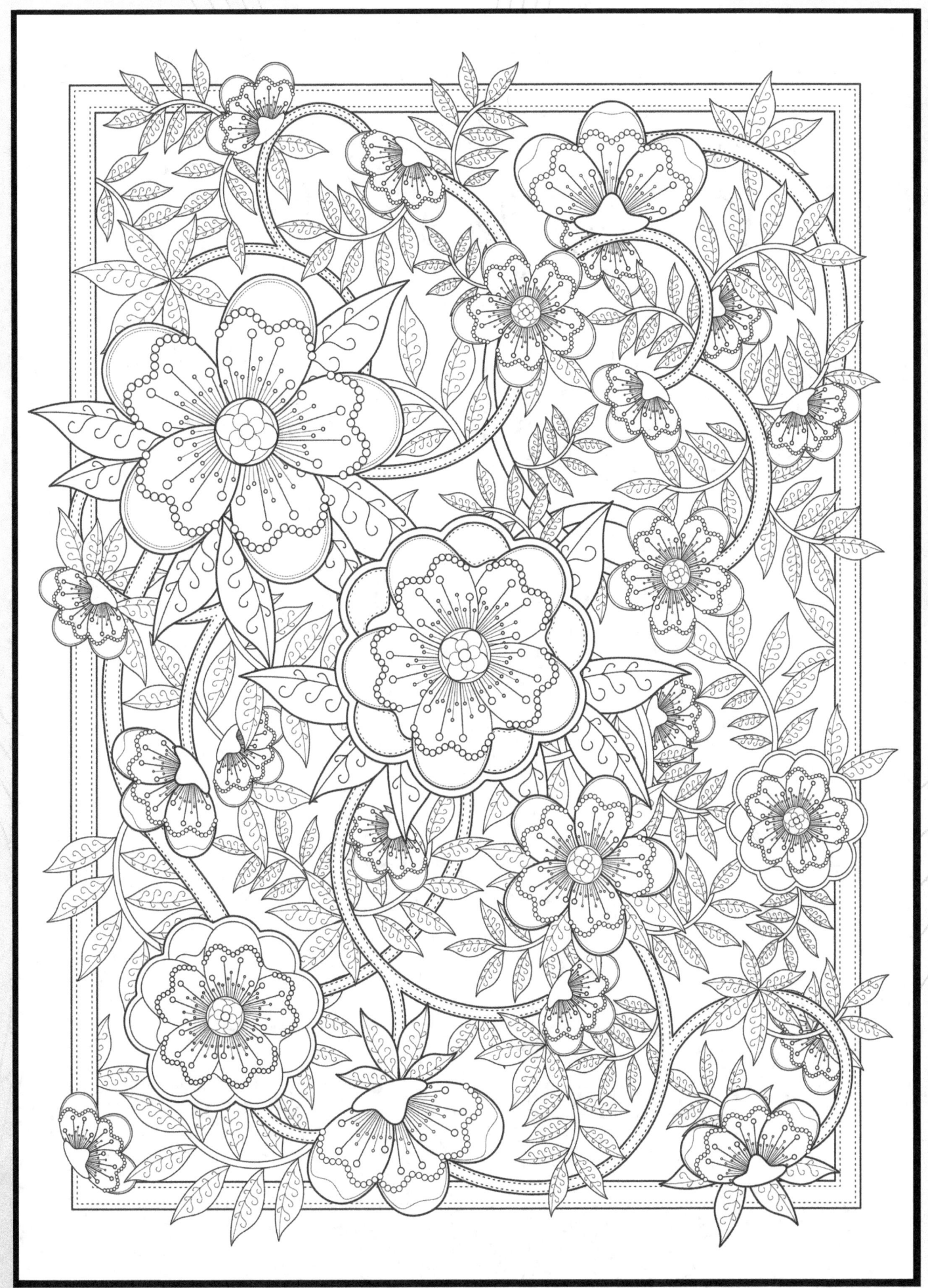

I've got 99 problems, but age ain't one

Find and trace all the numbers 7

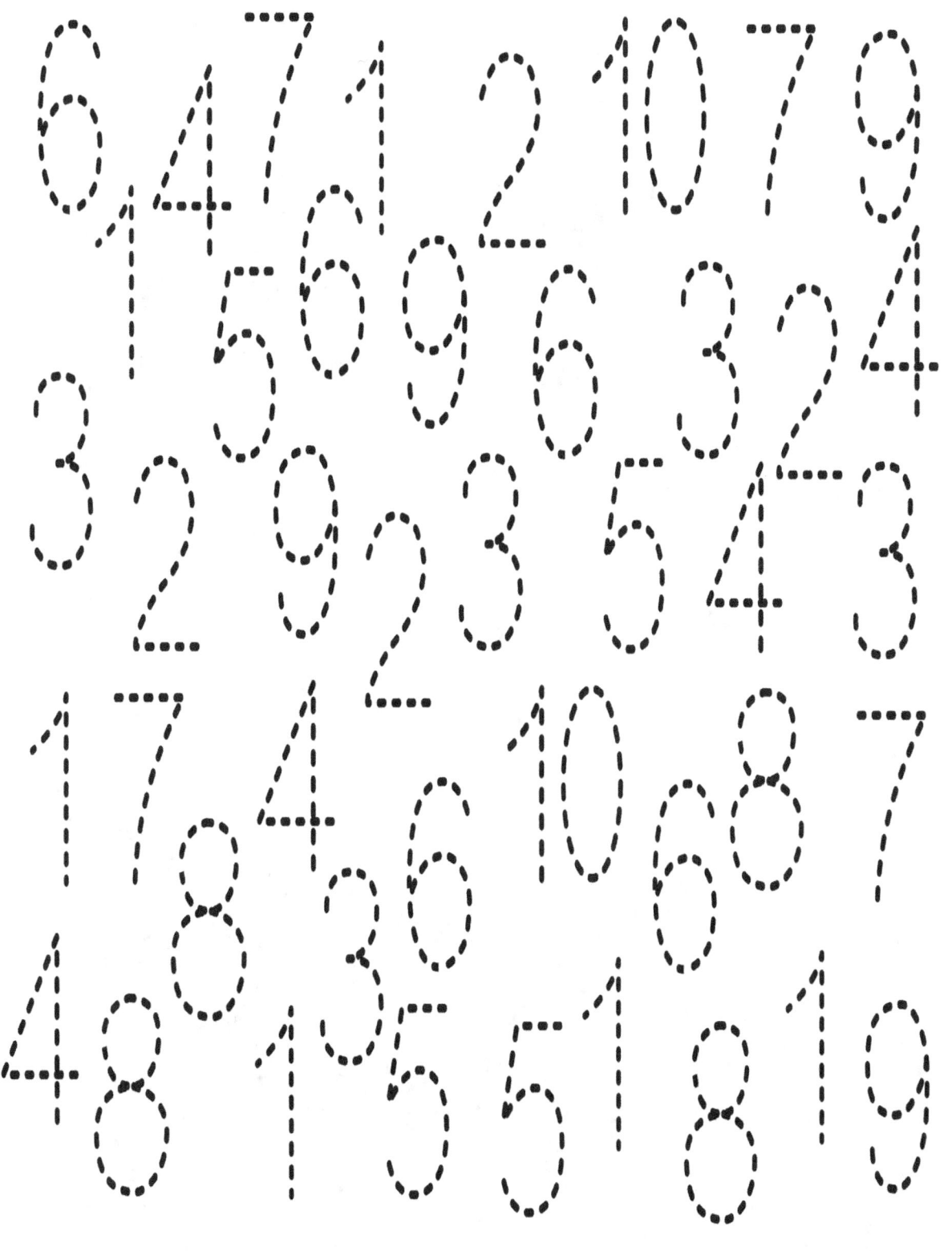

Connect the dots

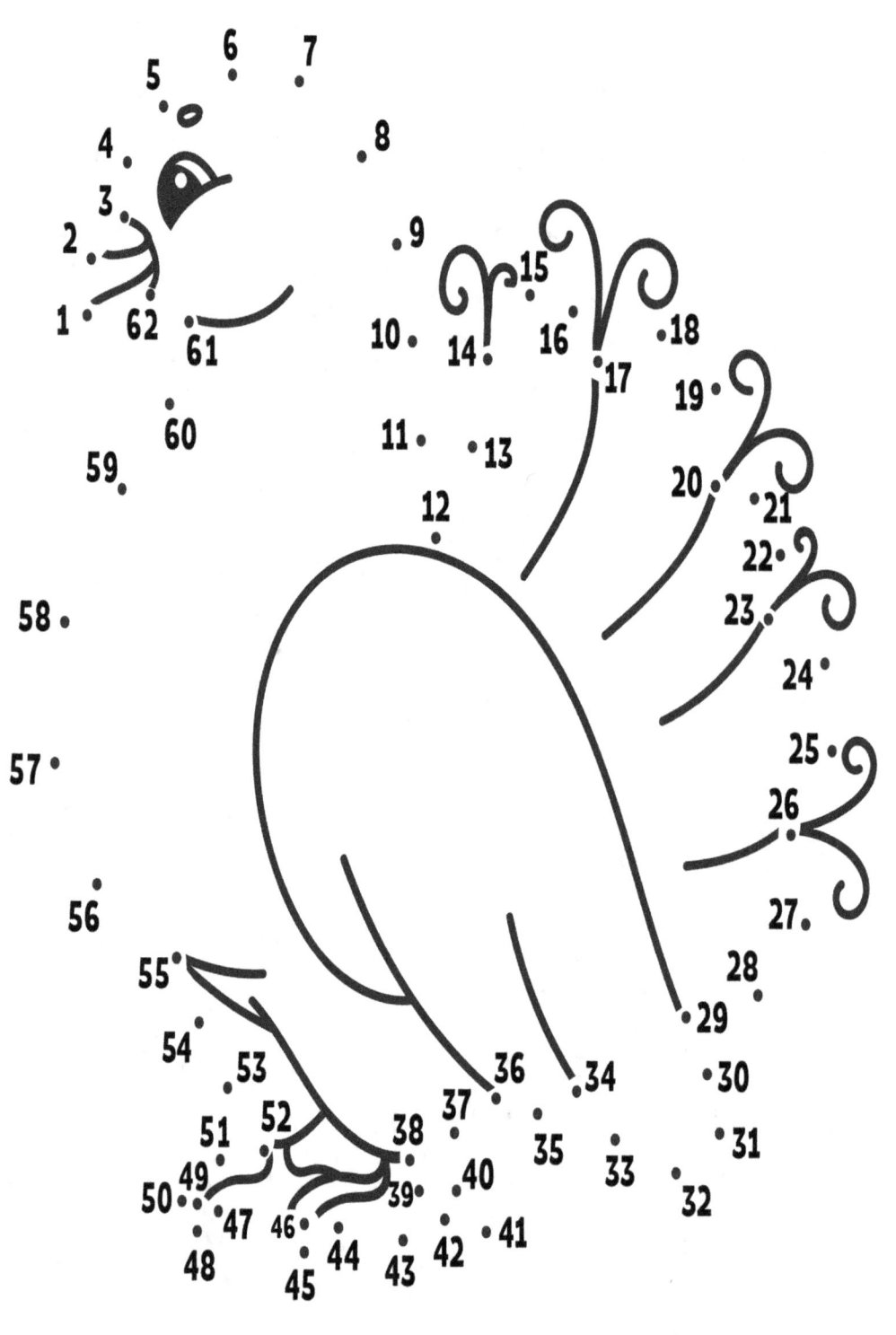

WORD SEARCH

FRIENDSHIP · LOVE · BEAUTY · FAMILY · HAPPINESS
MAN · WOMAN · GRAND · FEELING · LIFE

```
B D N A R G W I G F Z A I B H
G T L Q H Y K Q M O A U D B Q
Z C C D Q B J J B D H I D B X
K L N G J B U W E B B M Z F O
Y E Y Y E H I L A E Q O K B W
V Y B L W H I K U F L C U R T
J I U I C A E N T I Z U D C F
H W N M U P R D Y L Q L N H E
R X A A C P F W J E M O U X E
N G M F J I N T G G N A M N L
Q Z O D P N B K A L Y H V M I
C L W J E E F P P O I R G V N
R U F S V S F L S V C H R U G
R F A A P S D Z N E M L O G P
O C N I N P I H S D N E I R F
```

Trace

I

Find and color I

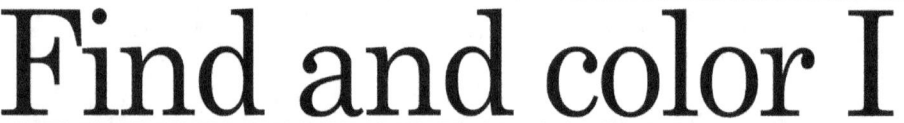

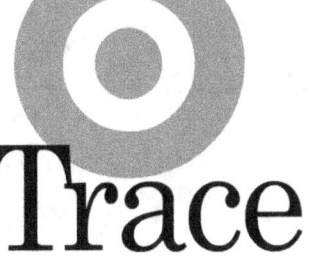

Trace

Find and color O

Q f e o o N o q
o G O O P Z p A
B i m s B O W
V o k o
o O Y T J O
o T R O q j o A
P O G U Q C O

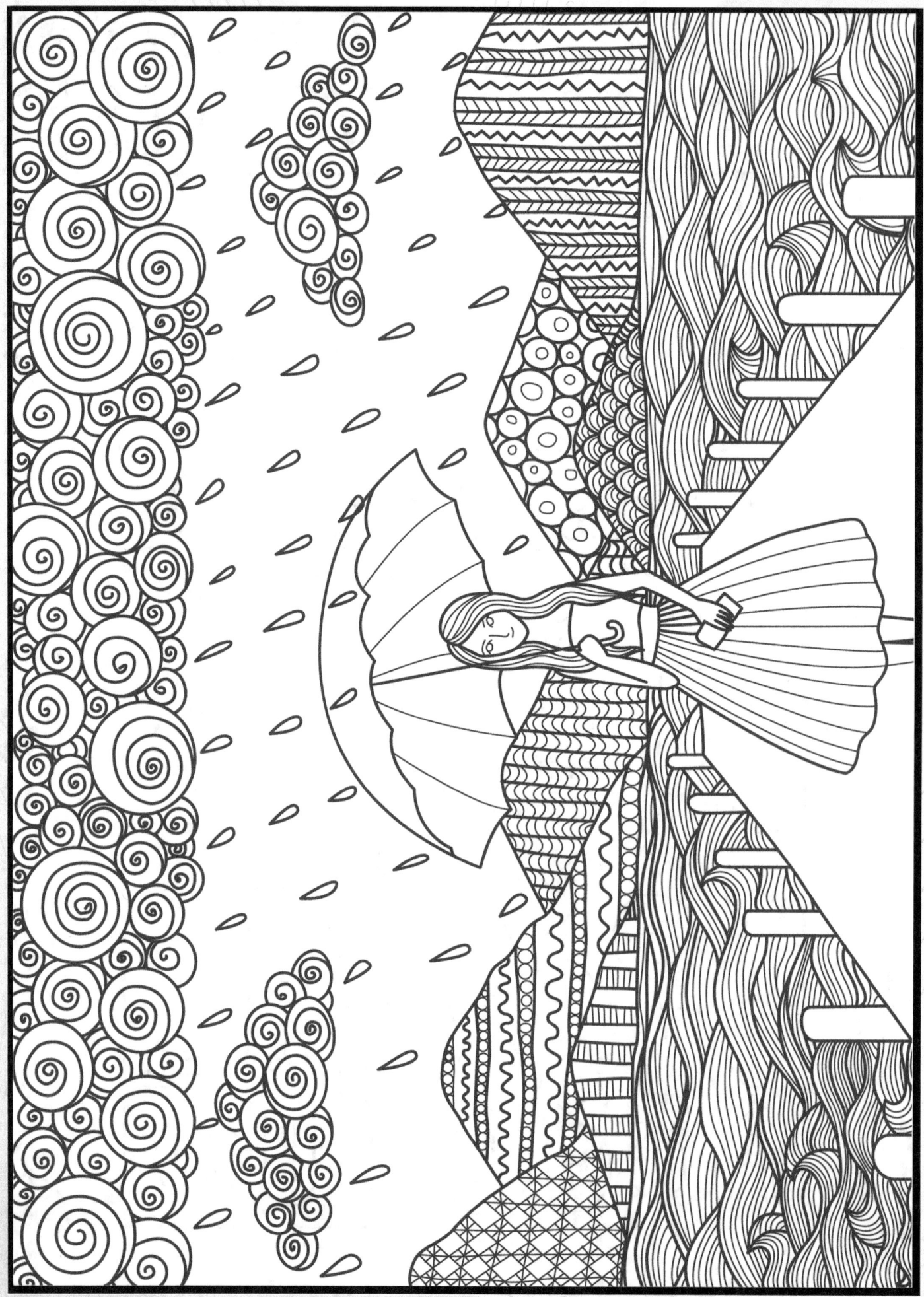

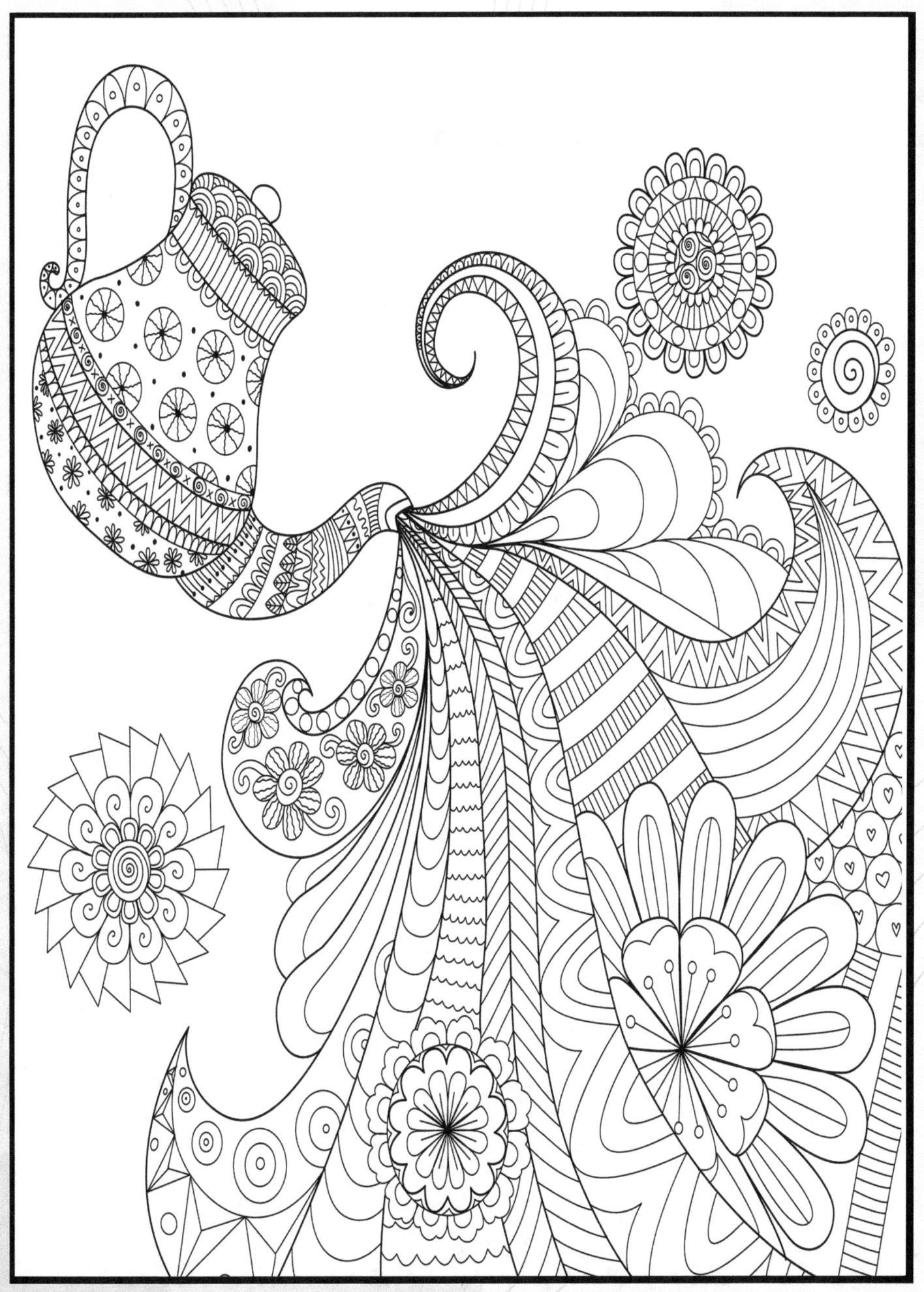

Subtraction

619 - 283	536 - 184	953 - 308	622 - 496
643 - 395	874 - 108	849 - 191	927 - 84
928 - 462	992 - 307	770 - 137	907 - 151
528 - 174	736 - 380	920 - 465	601 - 455

RIDDLES

1.- I'm tall when I'm young, and I'm short when I'm old. What am I?

2.- VWhat month of the year has 28 days?

3.- What is full of holes but still holds water?

4.- What can you break, even if you never pick it up or touch it?

5.- I shave every day, but my beard stays the same. What am I?

6.- The more of this there is, the less you see. What is it?

7.- What can you keep after giving to someone?

8.- What goes up but never comes down?

Solutions:

1.- A candle 2.- All of them 3.- A sponge 4.- A promise
5.- A barber 6.- Darkness 7.- Your word 8.- Your age

Trace the shapes

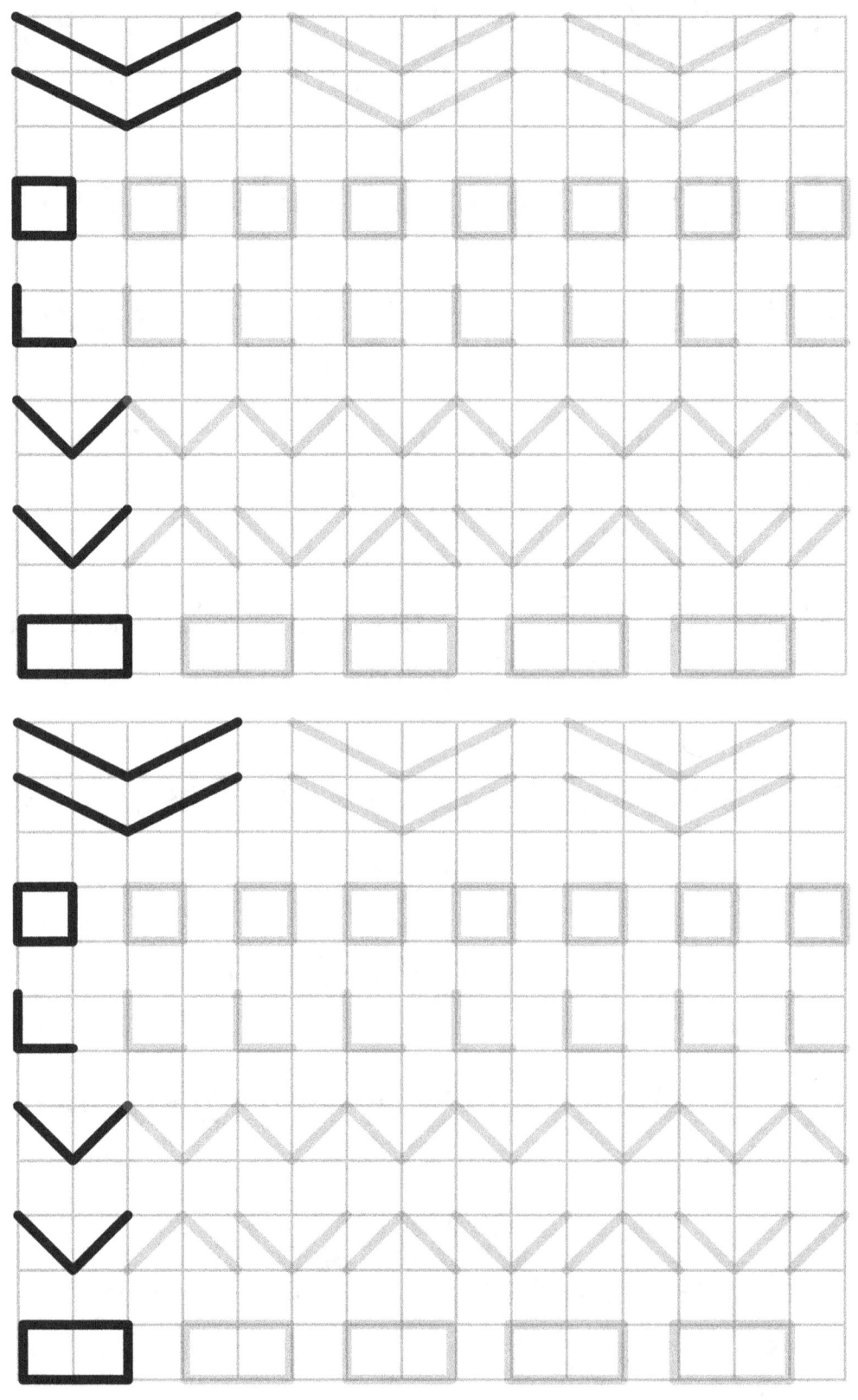

 Multiplication

351 x63	334 x39	477 x91	734 x75
730 x39	197 x47	659 x58	194 x87
277 x22	638 x64	992 x31	949 x17
521 x38	575 x71	254 x27	162 x84

5

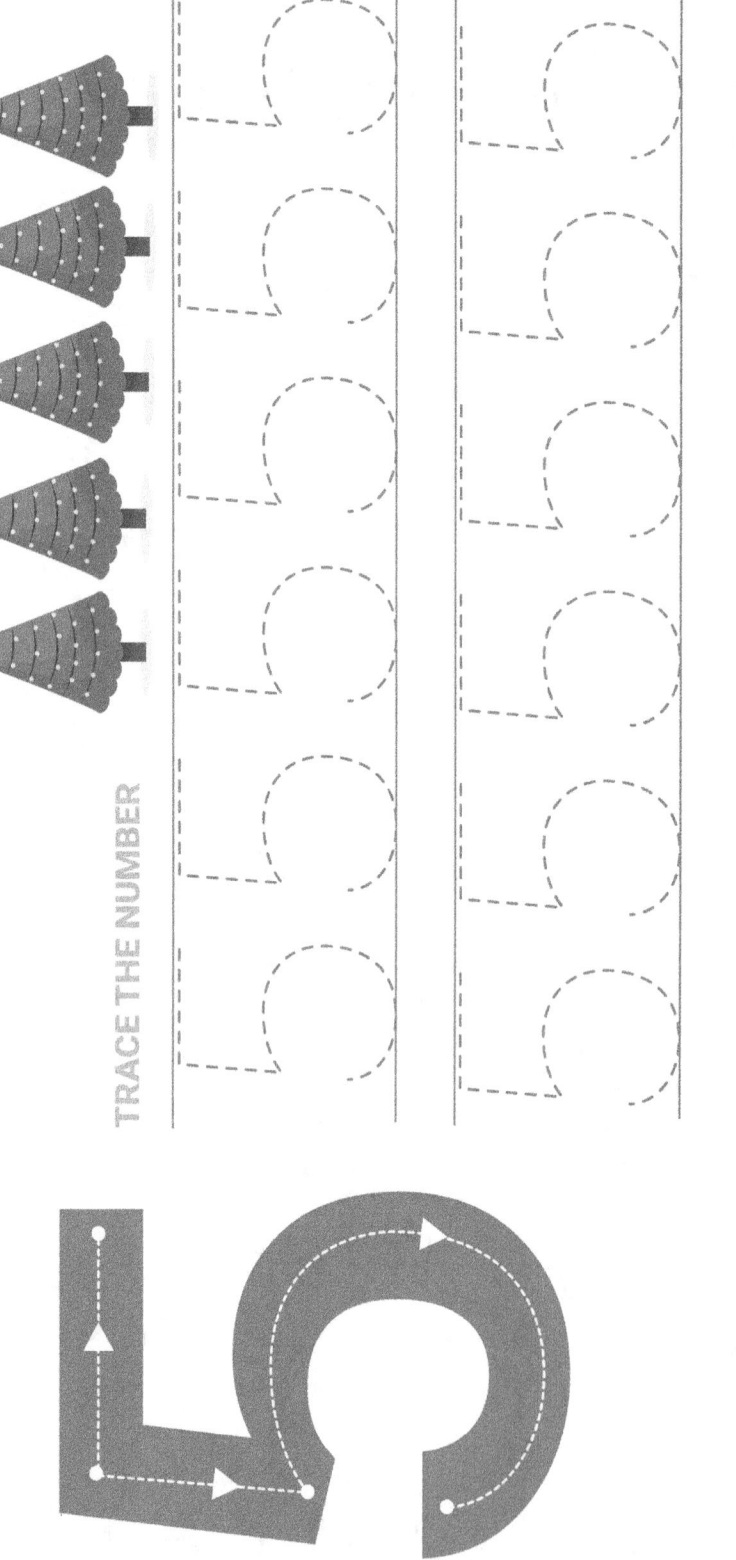

TRACE THE NUMBER

CIRCLE ALL THE NUMBER FIVE

1 2 3 4 5
2 3 1 1 5
5 2 4 3 1
5 1 4 3

CLOLOR FIVE CIRCLES

FIVE

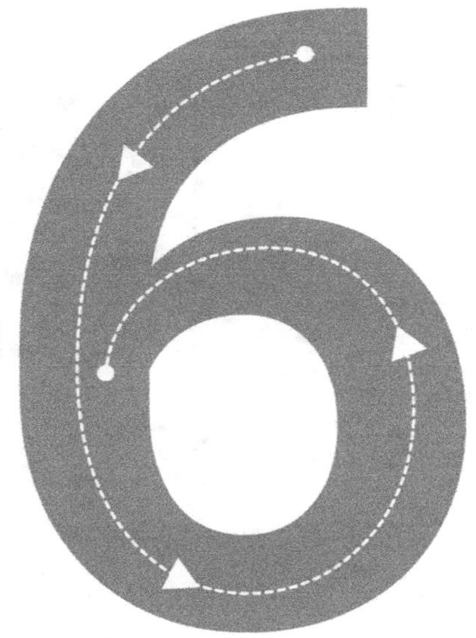

TRACE THE NUMBER

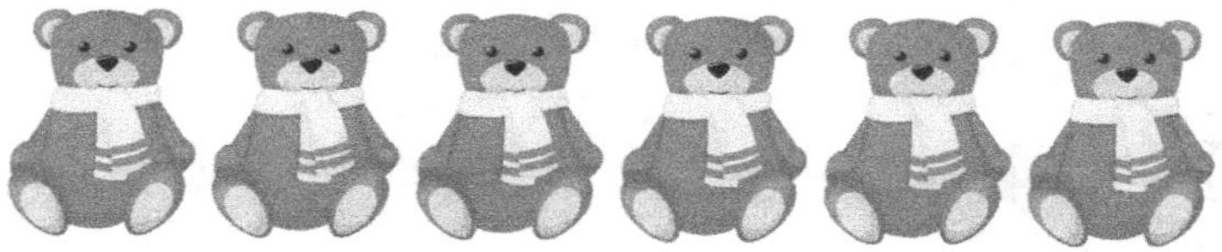

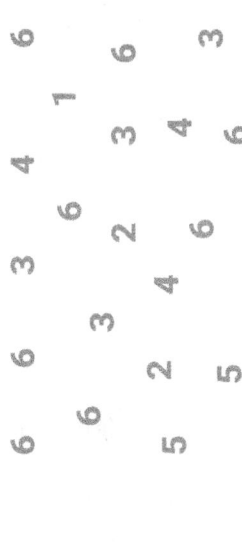

CIRCLE ALL THE NUMBER SIX

6 6 3 4 6 5
6 3 6 3 6 3
5 2 4 4 6
5 6

CLOLOR SIX CIRCLES

SIX

Finish the drawing and color

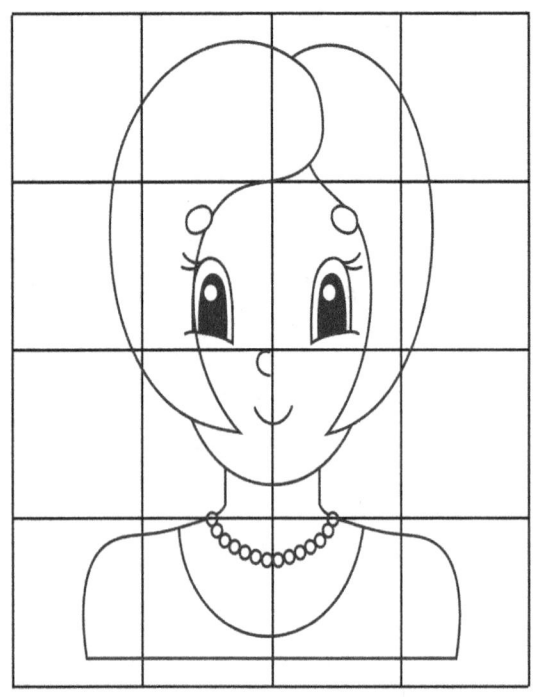 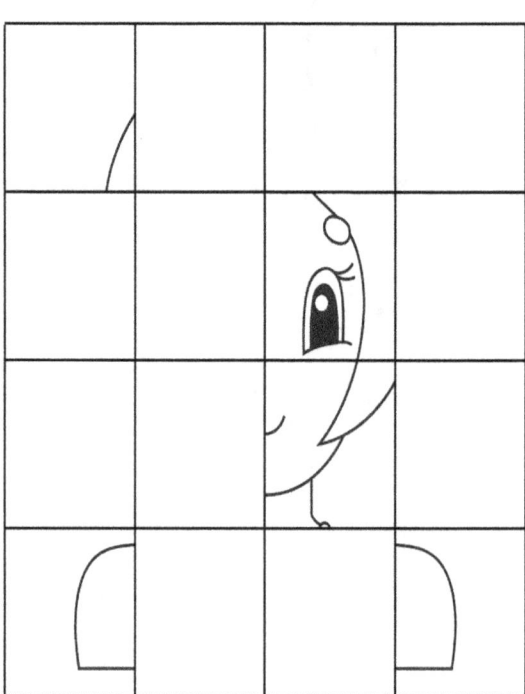

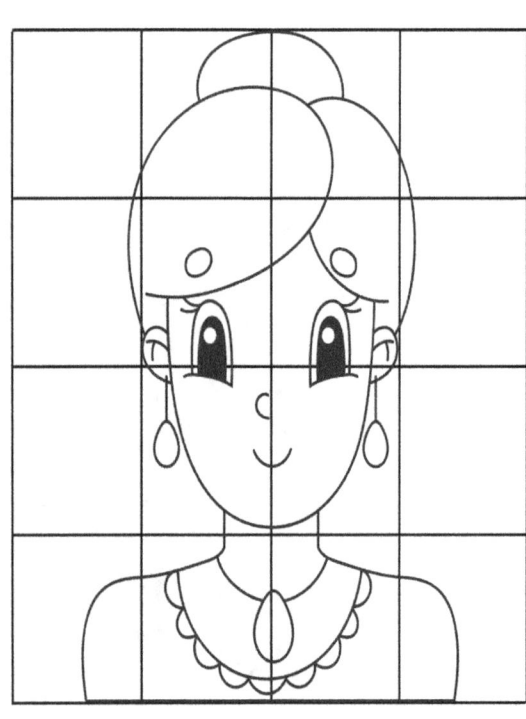 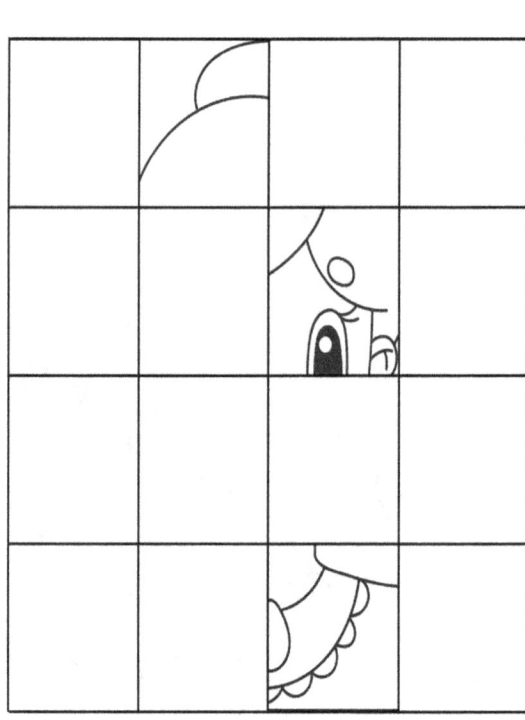

Complete the fractions

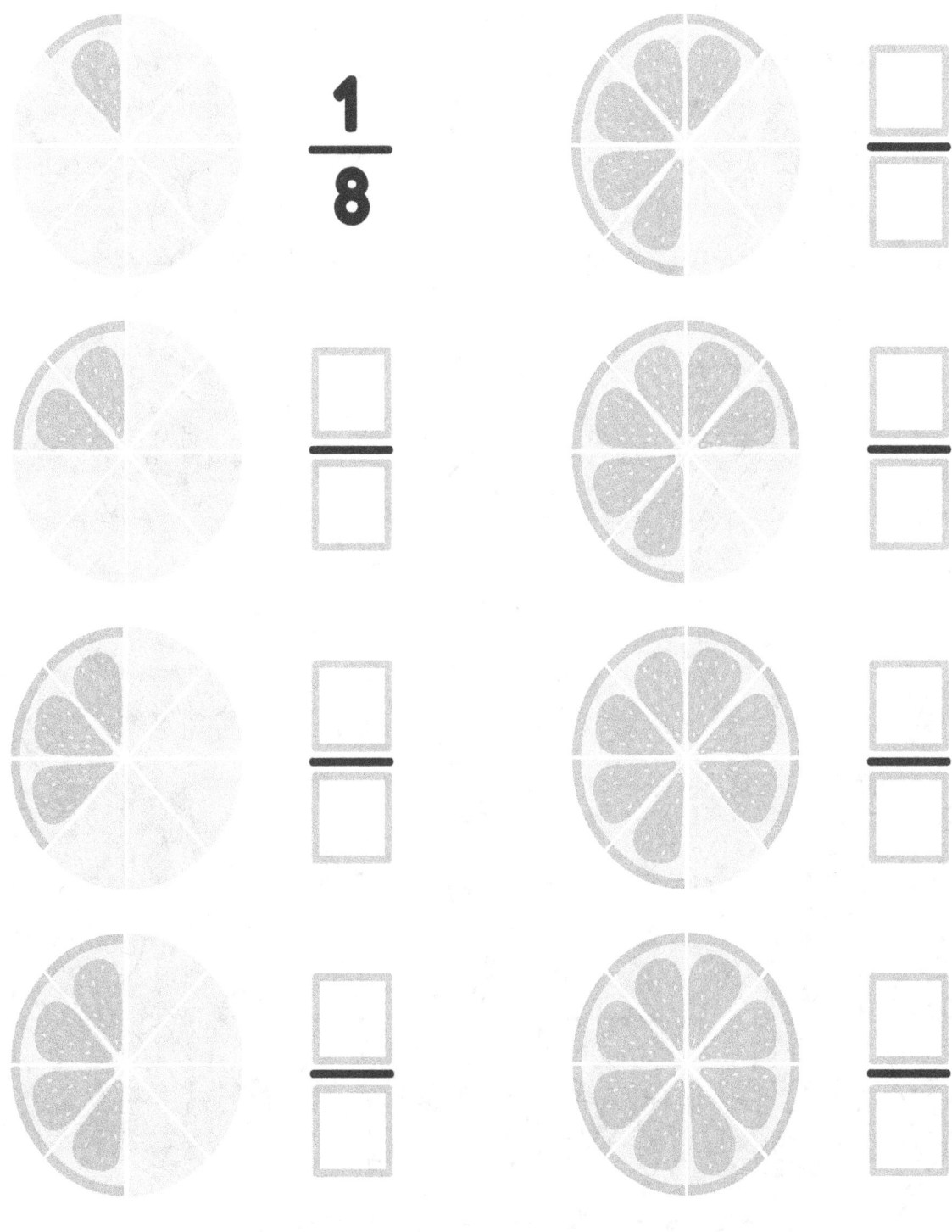

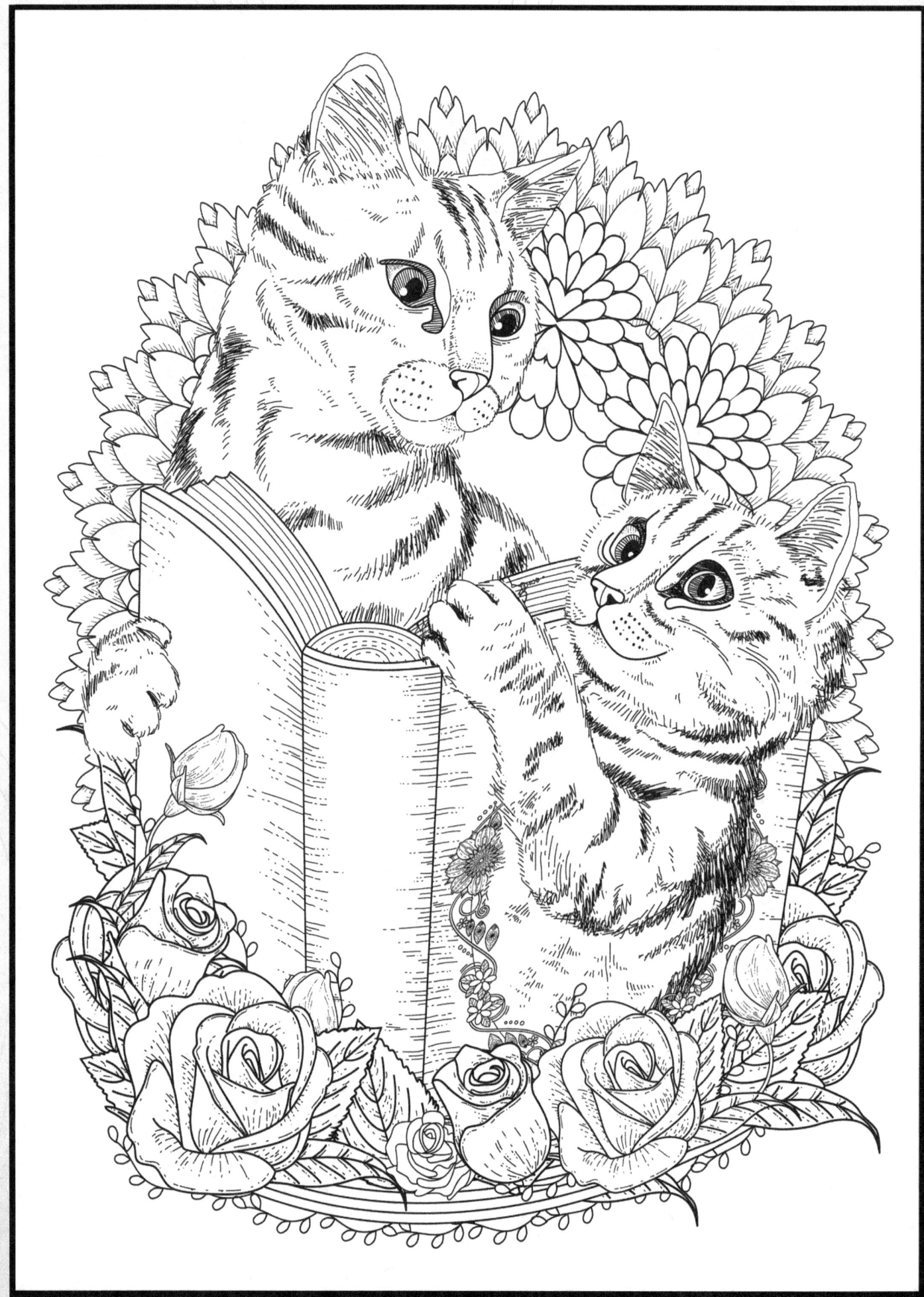

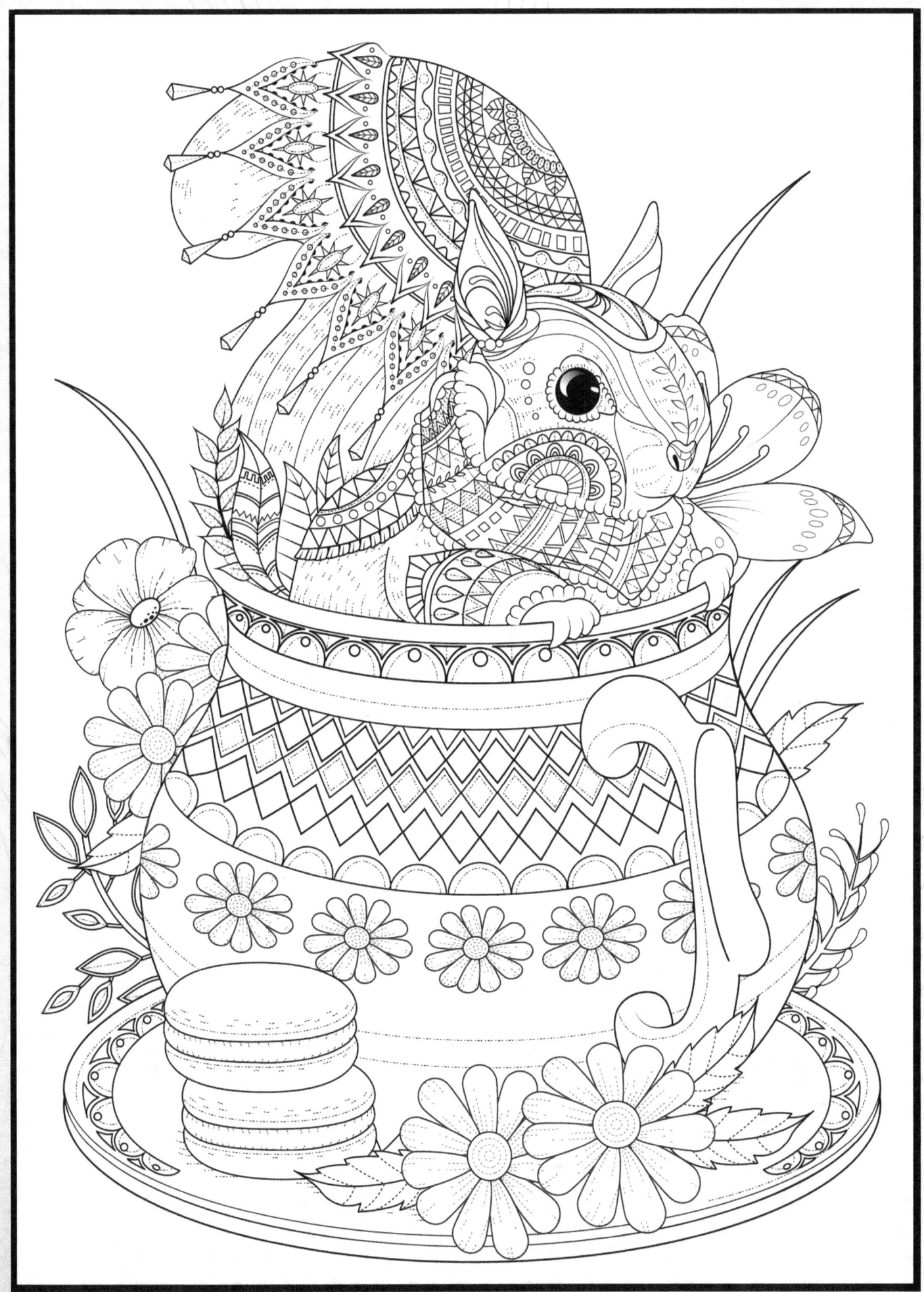

What time is it?

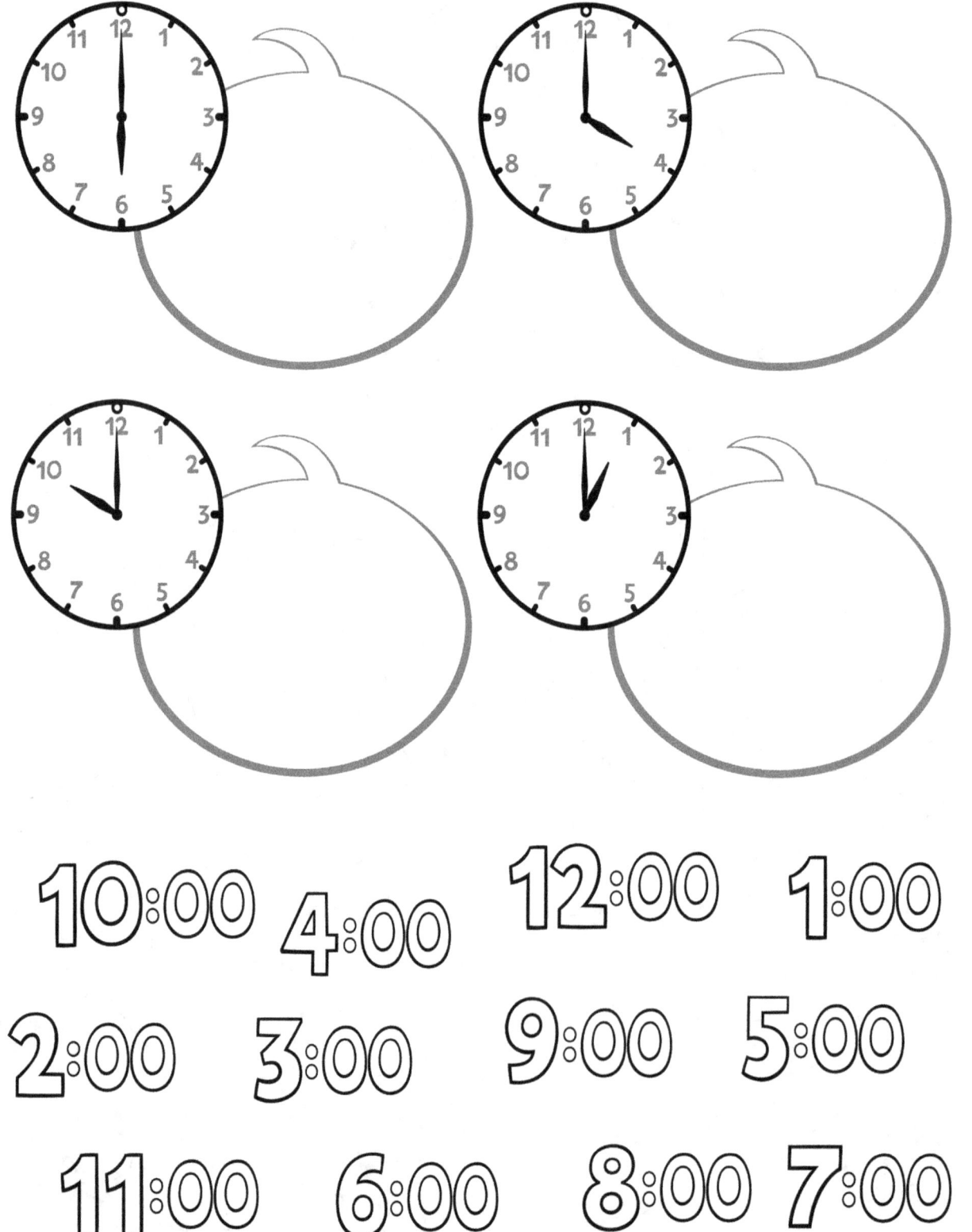

Trace with me

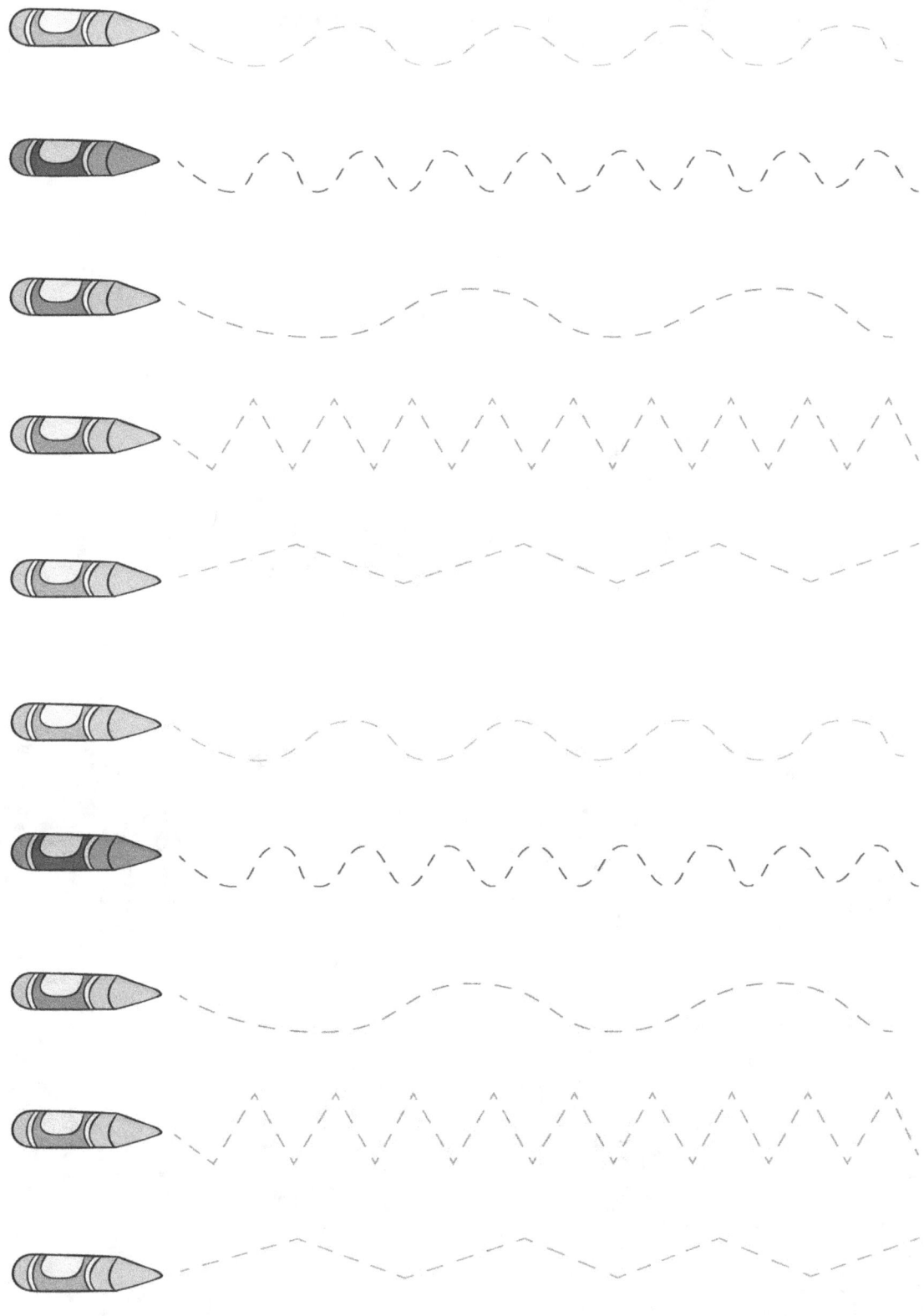

What is the name of each instrument?

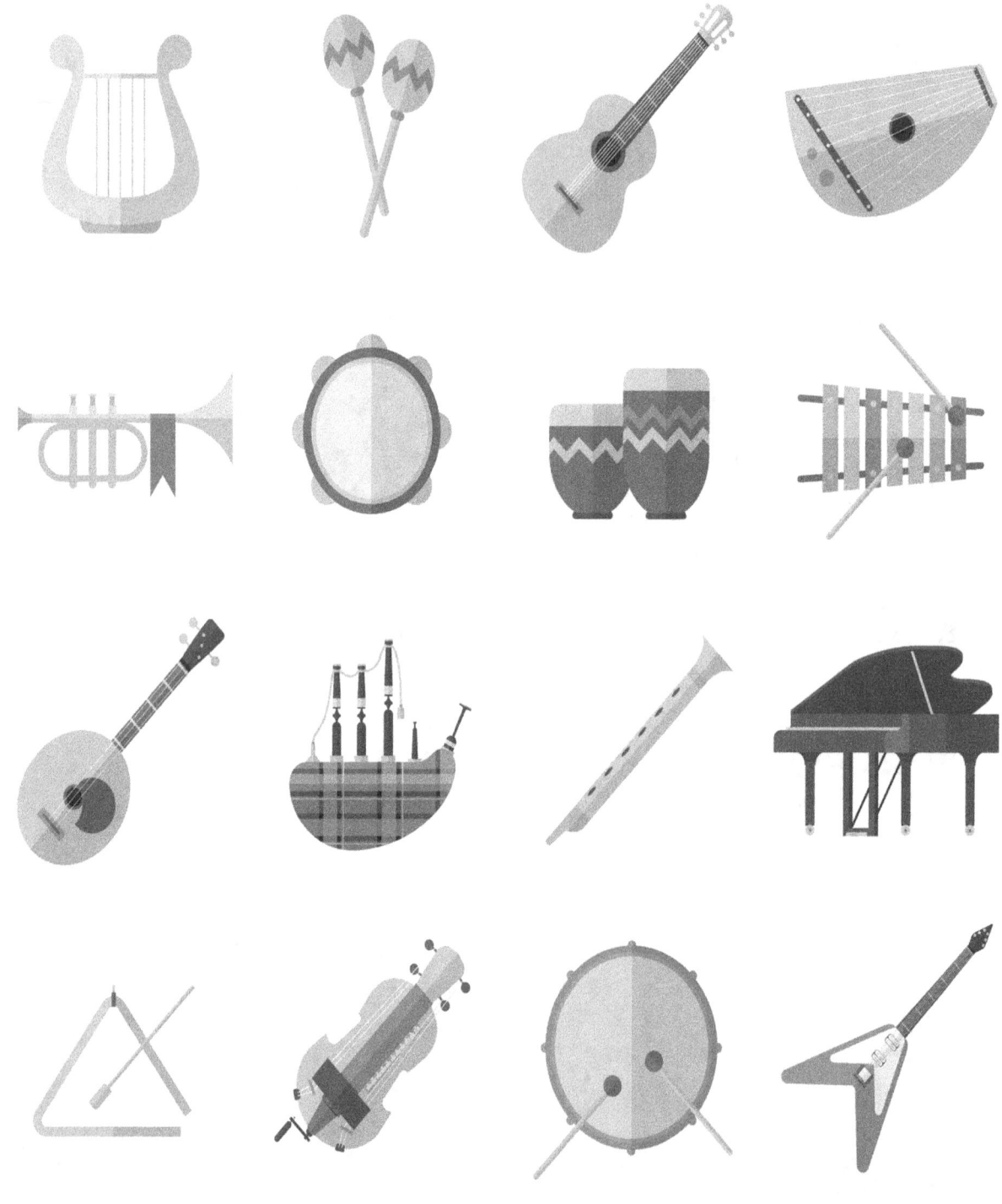

Paint each square
a different color

 Multiplication

206 x7	327 x6	700 x1	449 x8
138 x4	677 x9	414 x7	151 x8
250 x9	248 x1	564 x5	458 x6
713 x6	897 x8	169 x8	615 x7

Let´s review calligraphy

To shine your brightest light is to be who you truly are

Happiness depends on your mindset and attitude

Smile more. Smiling can make you and others happy

Let's review calligraphy

Be mindful. Be grateful. Be positive. Be true. Be kind.

Accept yourself, love yourself, and keep moving forward

Be brave to stand for what you believe in even if you stand alone

Get to number 16 going through the numbers in order

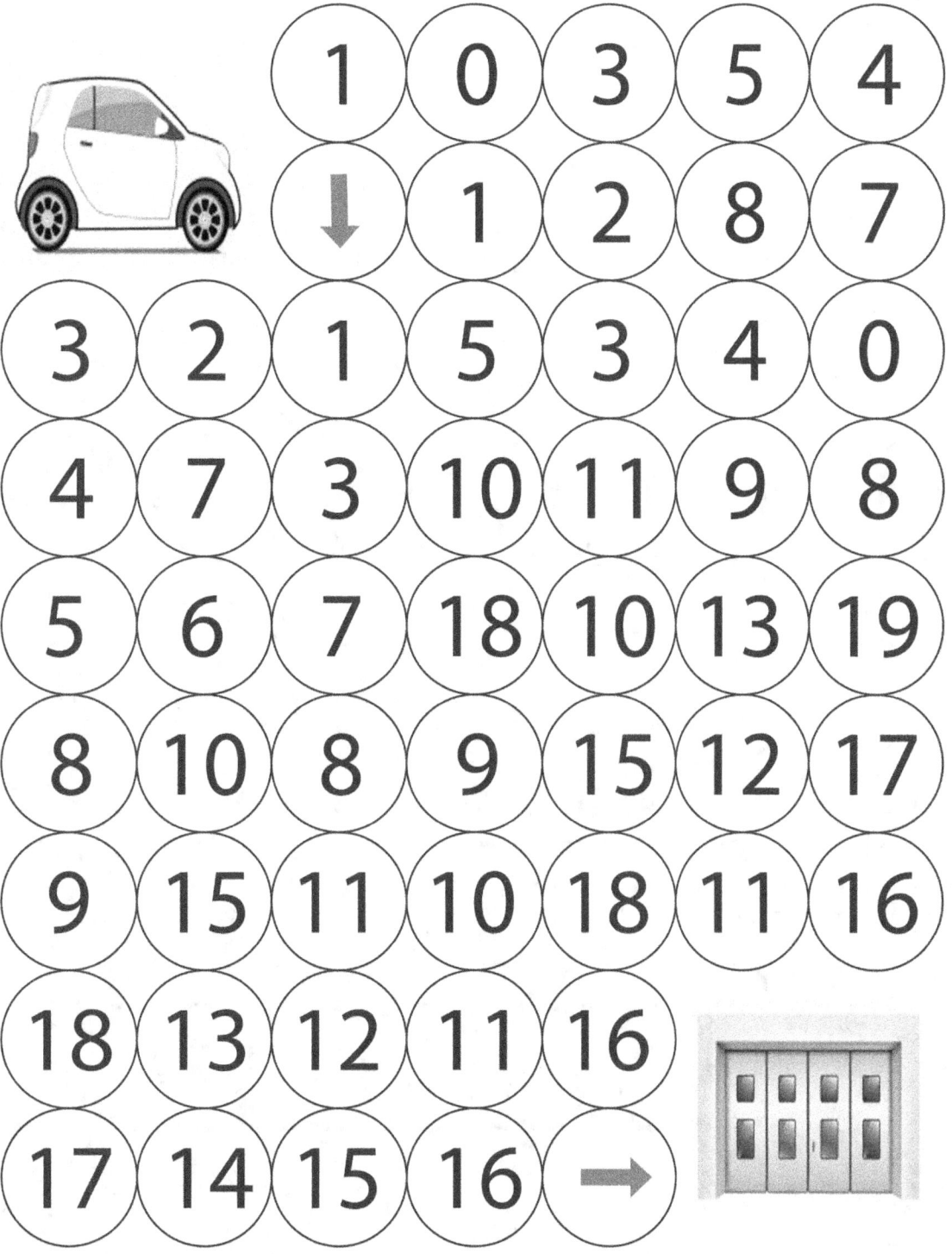

It always seems impossible until it is done

How many cows are looking each side?

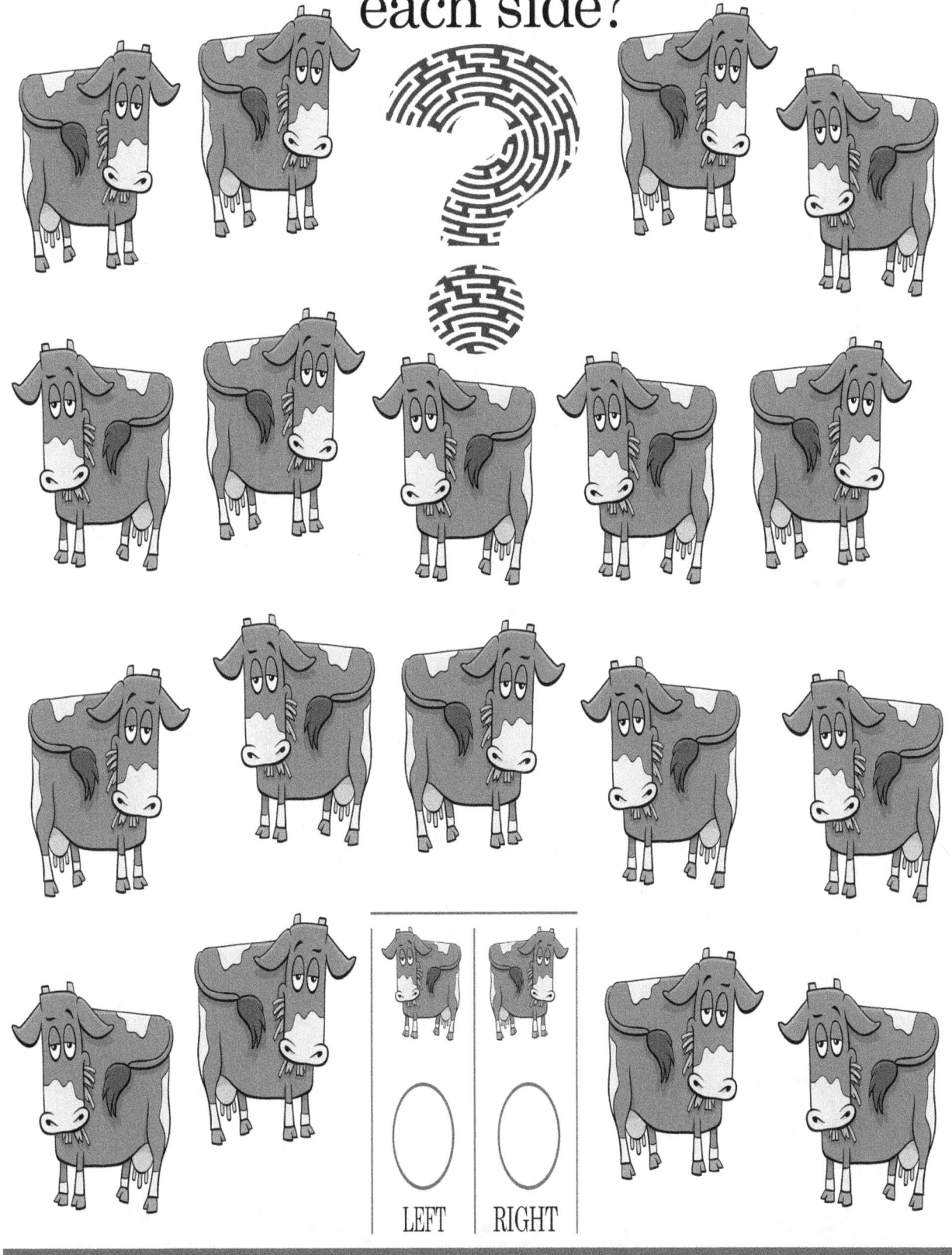

LEFT   RIGHT

Trace the shapes

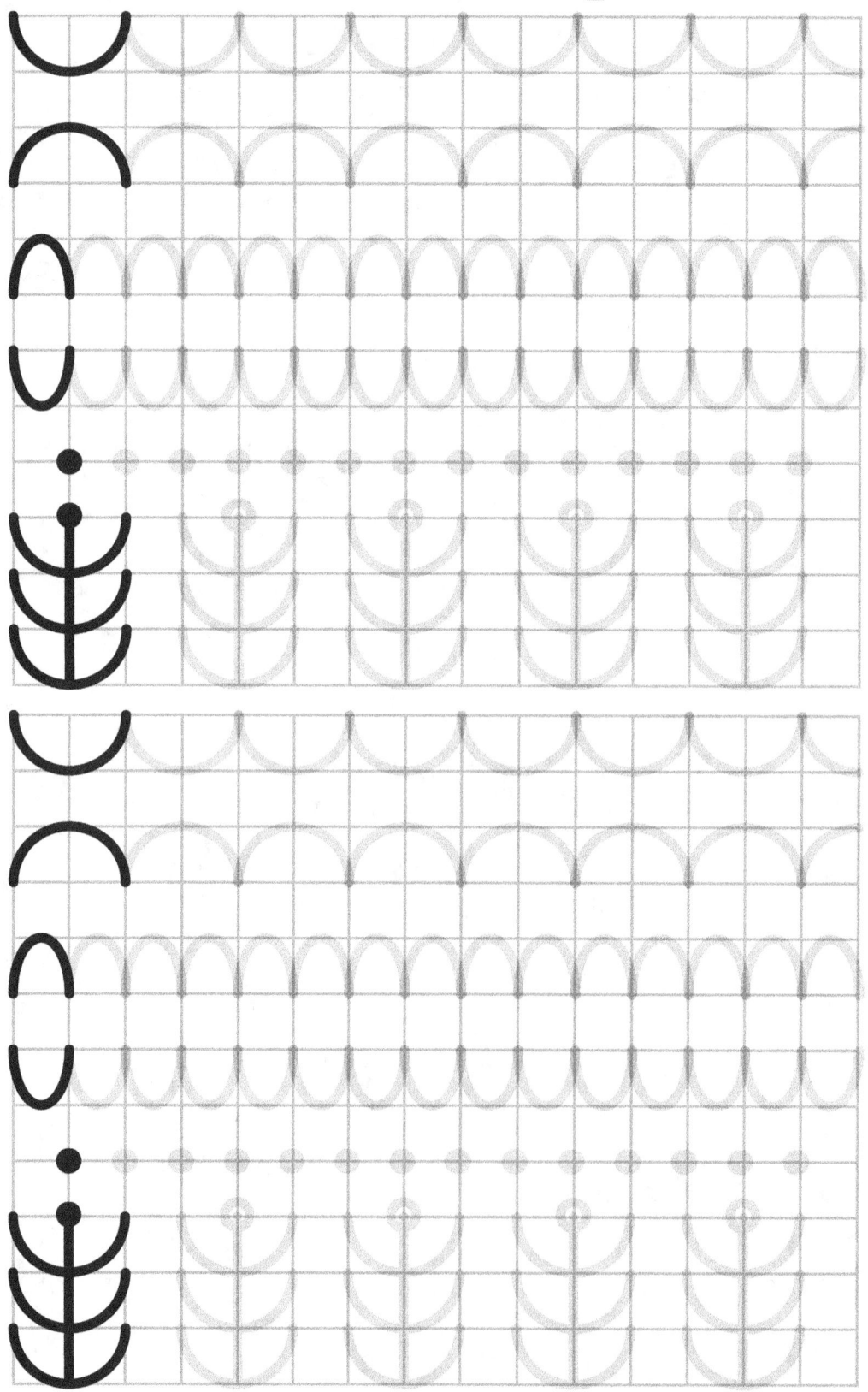

How many floors does each building ?

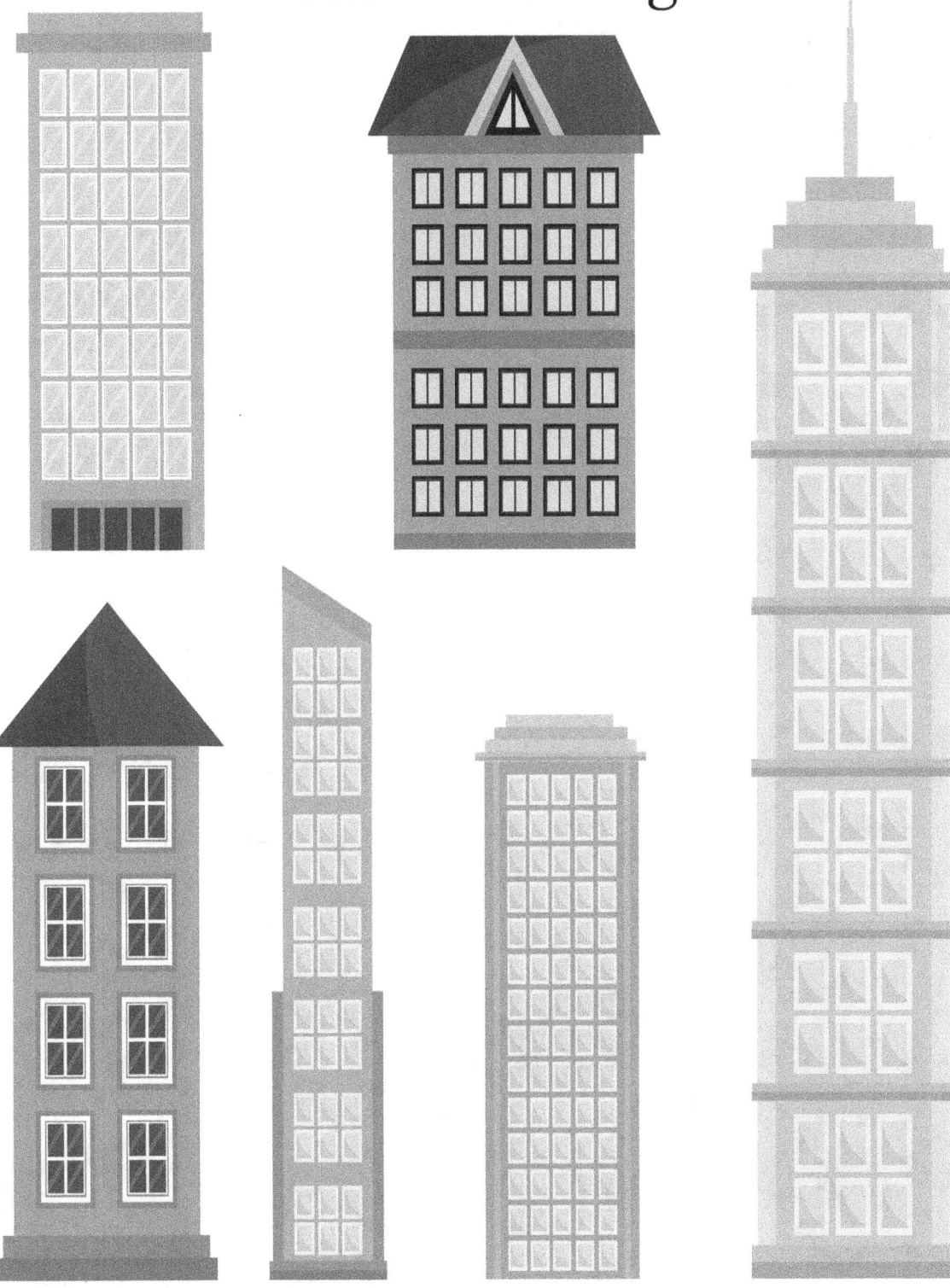

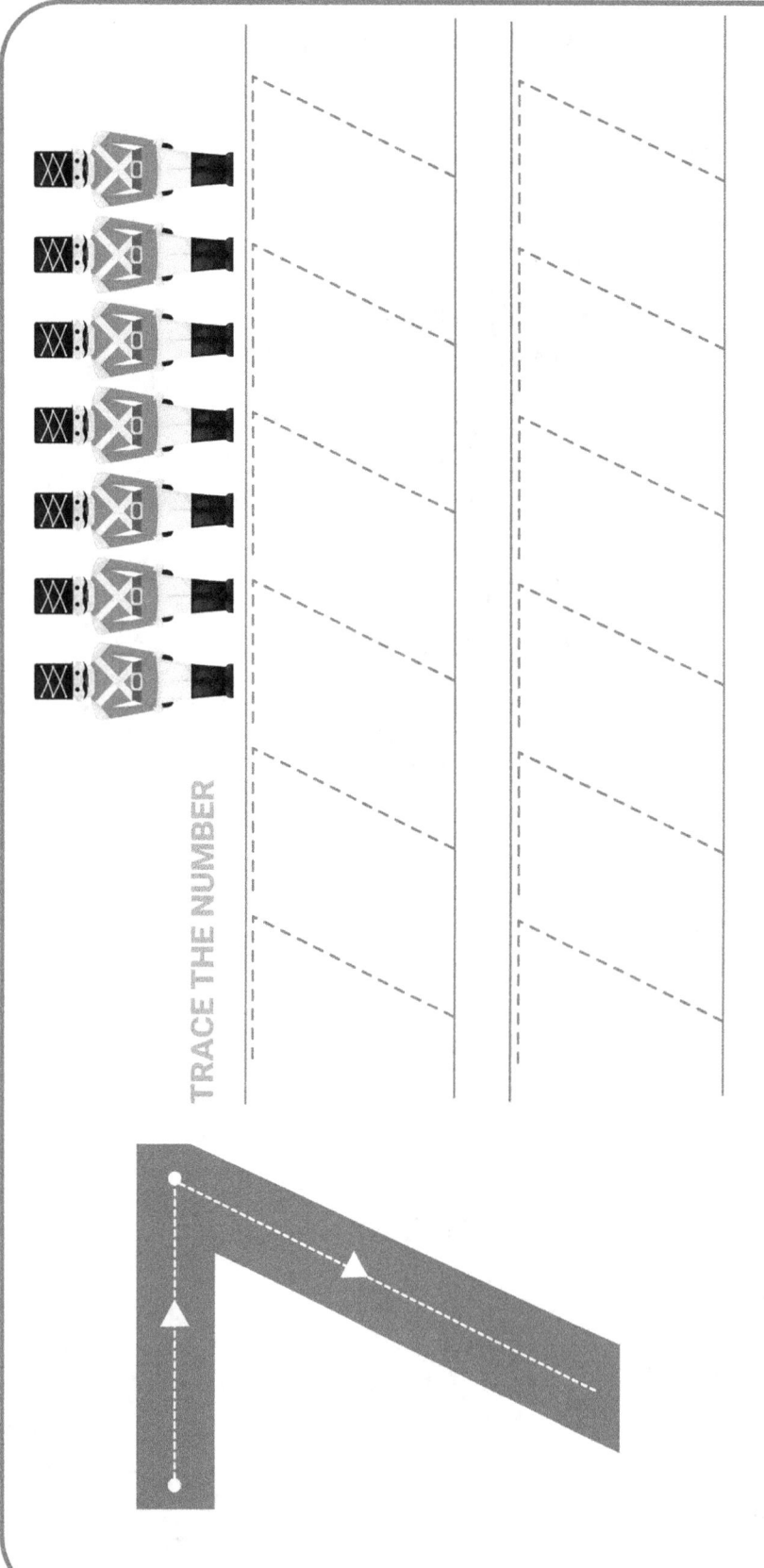

TRACE THE NUMBER

CIRCLE ALL THE NUMBER SEVEN

6	6	3	4	7	5
7	3	6	1	7	7
5	2	7	3	6	3
7	7	6	4	7	

CLOLOR SEVEN CIRCLES

SEVEN

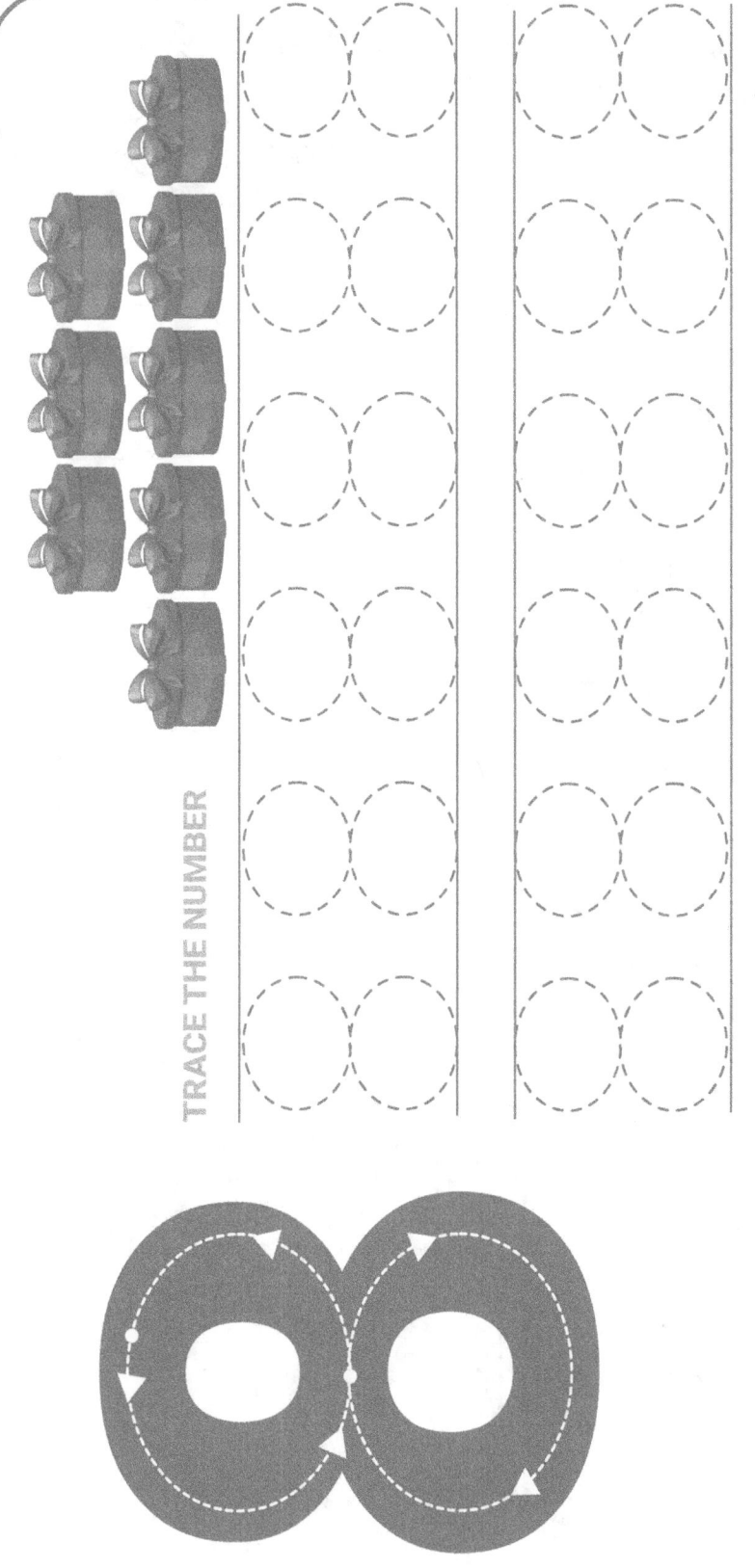

TRACE THE NUMBER

CIRCLE ALL THE NUMBER EIGHT

6	8	3	8	7	5
1	3	6	1	8	1
4	2	8	7	4	8
	7	5			

CLOLOR EIGHT CIRCLES

EIGHT

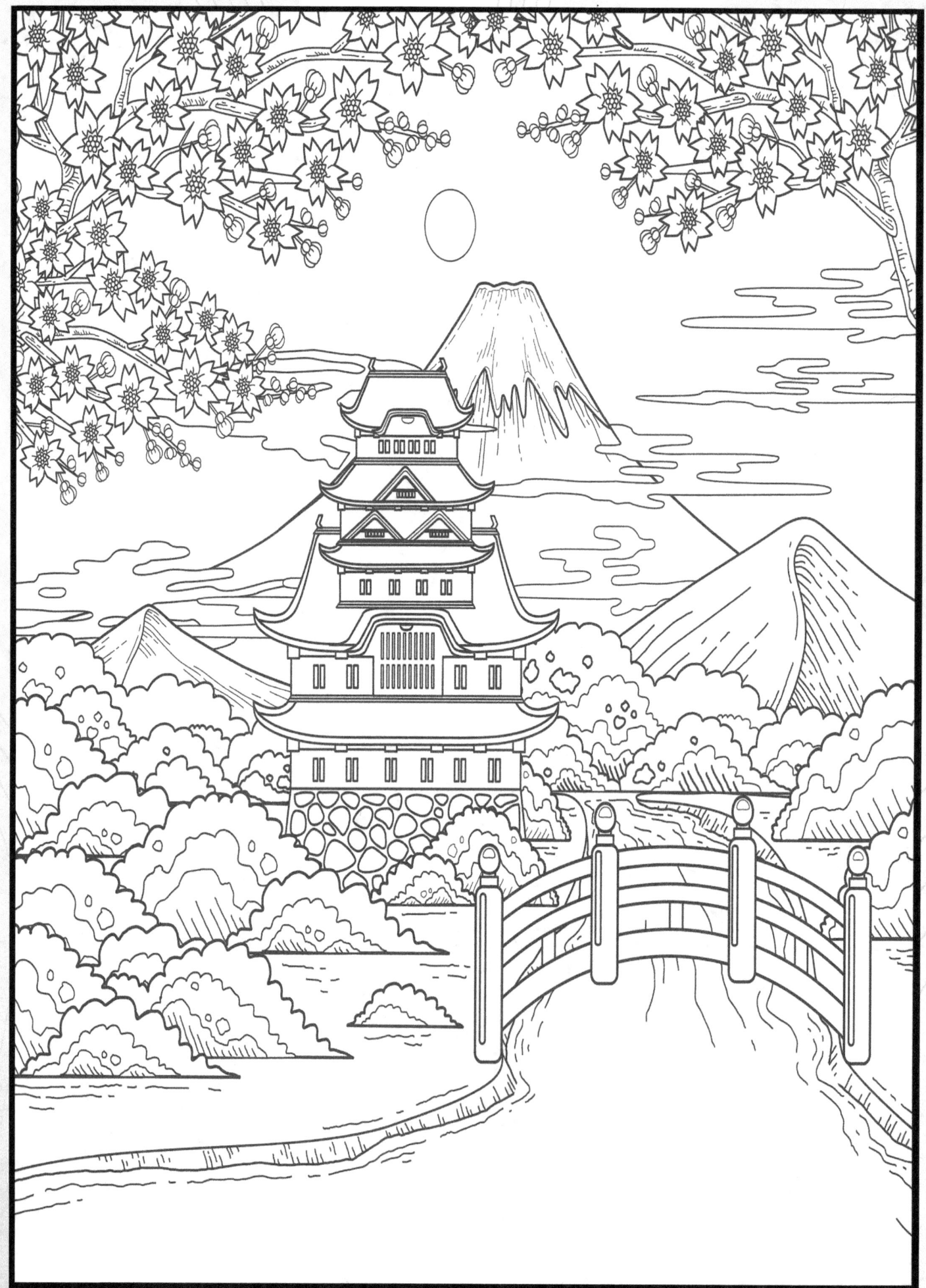

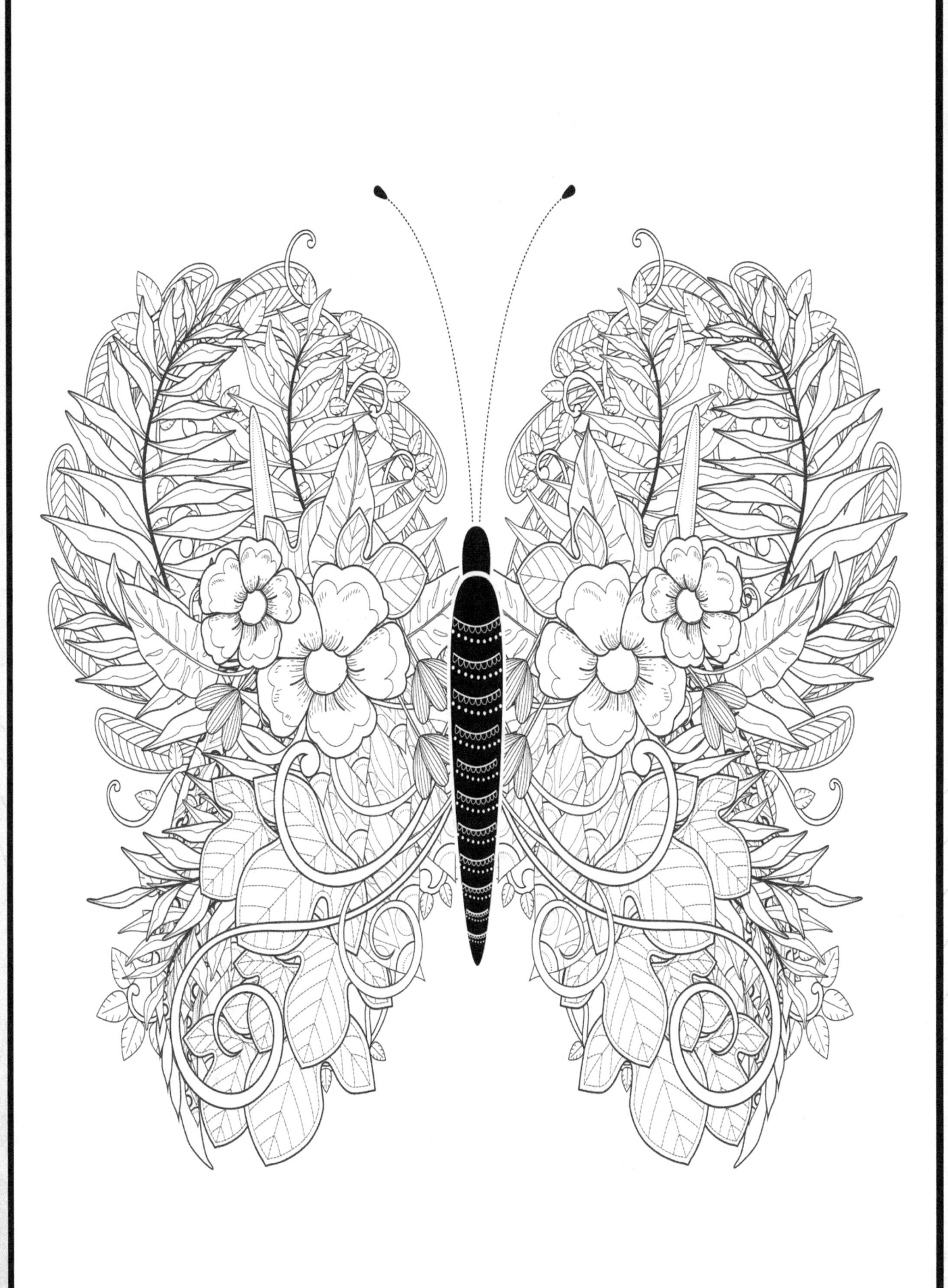

What activity does each picture show?

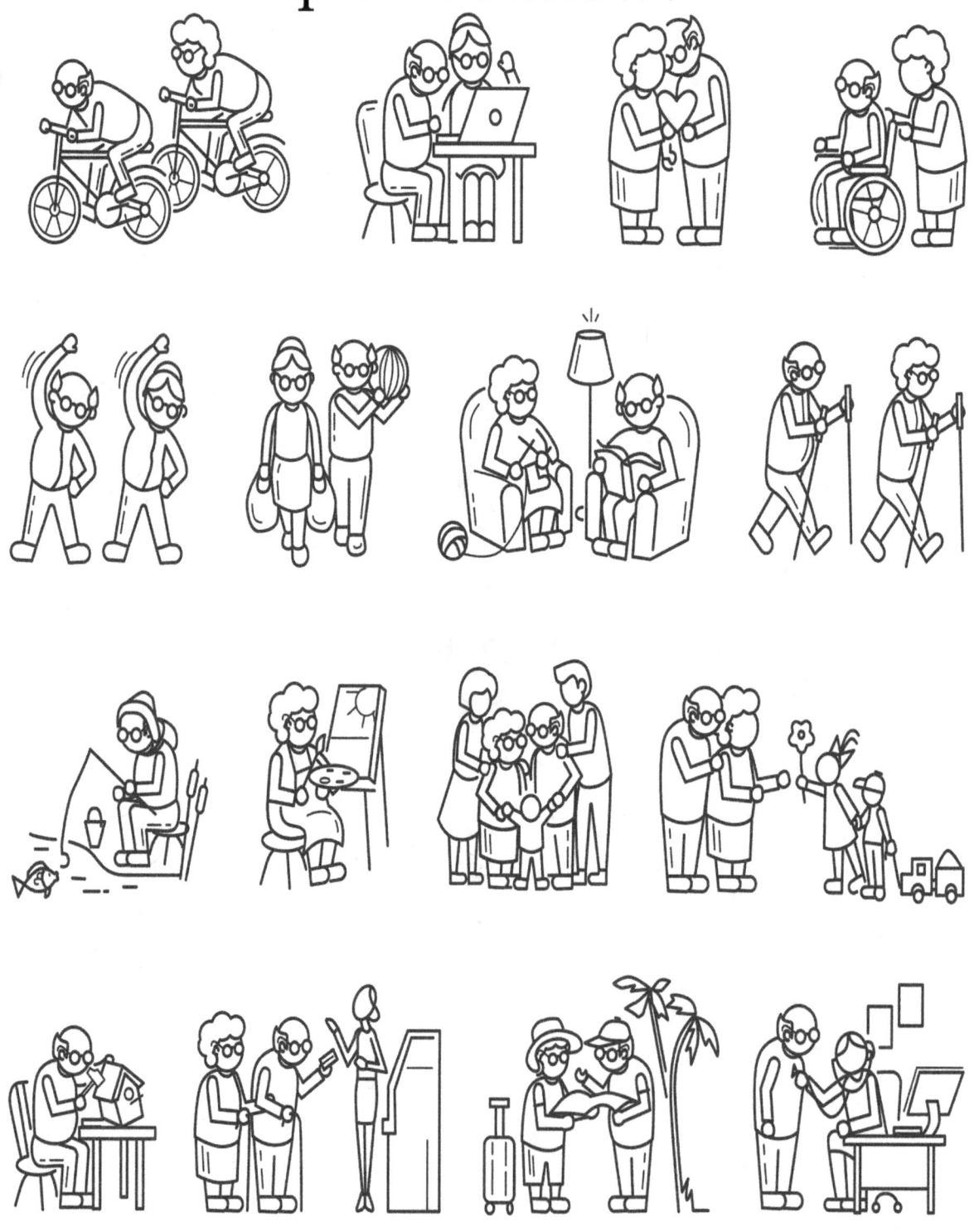

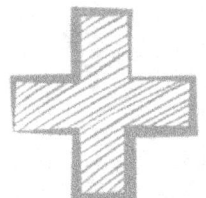 Sums

$$+\ \begin{matrix}25\\35\end{matrix}\qquad +\ \begin{matrix}37\\08\end{matrix}\qquad +\ \begin{matrix}73\\70\end{matrix}\qquad +\ \begin{matrix}17\\08\end{matrix}\qquad +\ \begin{matrix}09\\09\end{matrix}\qquad +\ \begin{matrix}71\\61\end{matrix}$$

$$+\ \begin{matrix}29\\16\end{matrix}\qquad +\ \begin{matrix}54\\80\end{matrix}\qquad +\ \begin{matrix}05\\29\end{matrix}\qquad +\ \begin{matrix}28\\49\end{matrix}\qquad +\ \begin{matrix}71\\73\end{matrix}\qquad +\ \begin{matrix}45\\05\end{matrix}$$

$$+\ \begin{matrix}35\\07\end{matrix}\qquad +\ \begin{matrix}36\\18\end{matrix}\qquad +\ \begin{matrix}61\\51\end{matrix}\qquad +\ \begin{matrix}19\\36\end{matrix}\qquad +\ \begin{matrix}92\\72\end{matrix}\qquad +\ \begin{matrix}47\\39\end{matrix}$$

$$+\ \begin{matrix}60\\84\end{matrix}\qquad +\ \begin{matrix}62\\54\end{matrix}\qquad +\ \begin{matrix}50\\52\end{matrix}\qquad +\ \begin{matrix}36\\19\end{matrix}\qquad +\ \begin{matrix}94\\60\end{matrix}\qquad +\ \begin{matrix}91\\70\end{matrix}$$

How many butterflies are there?

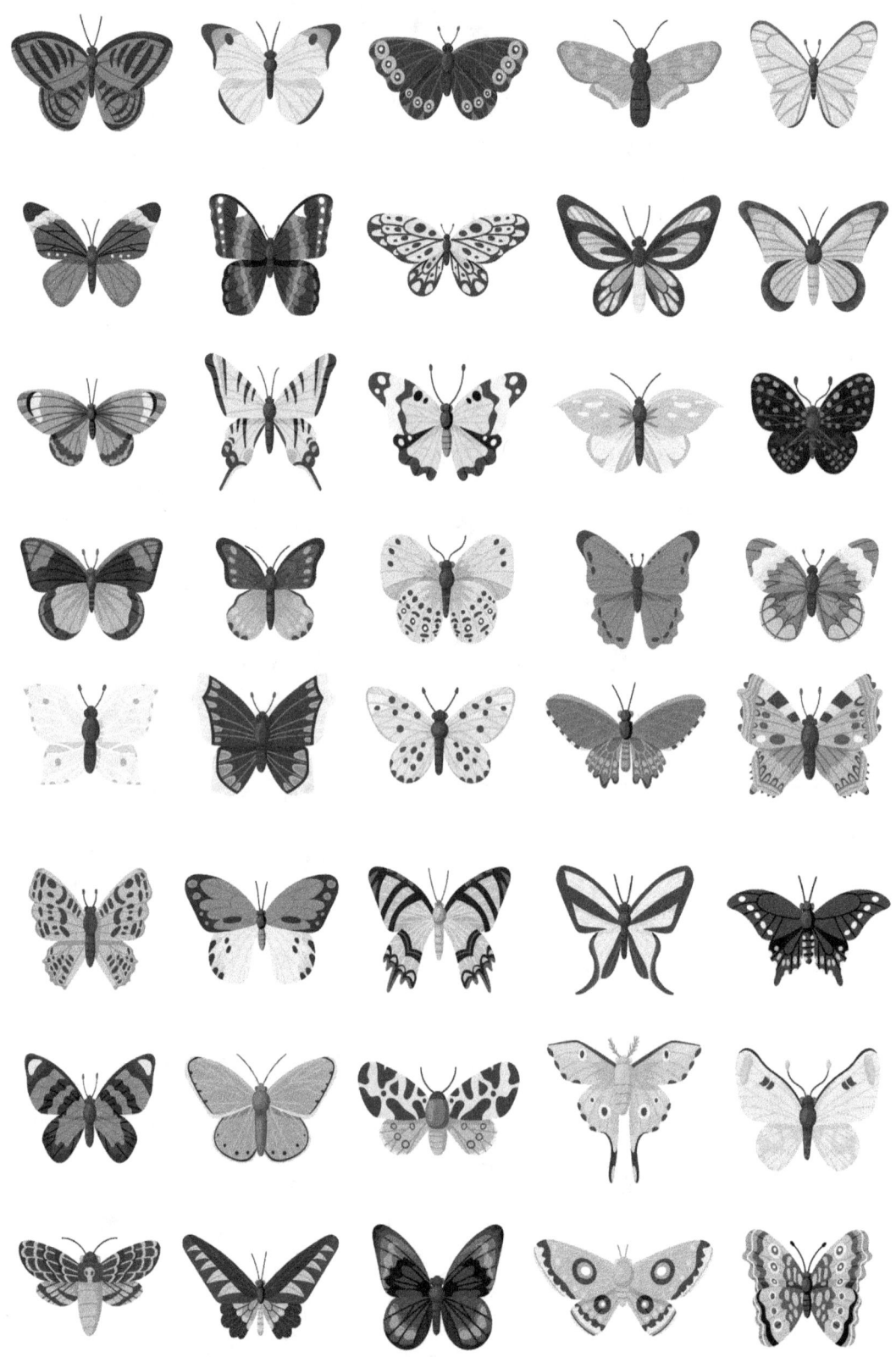

How many clothes are hanging on the clothesline?

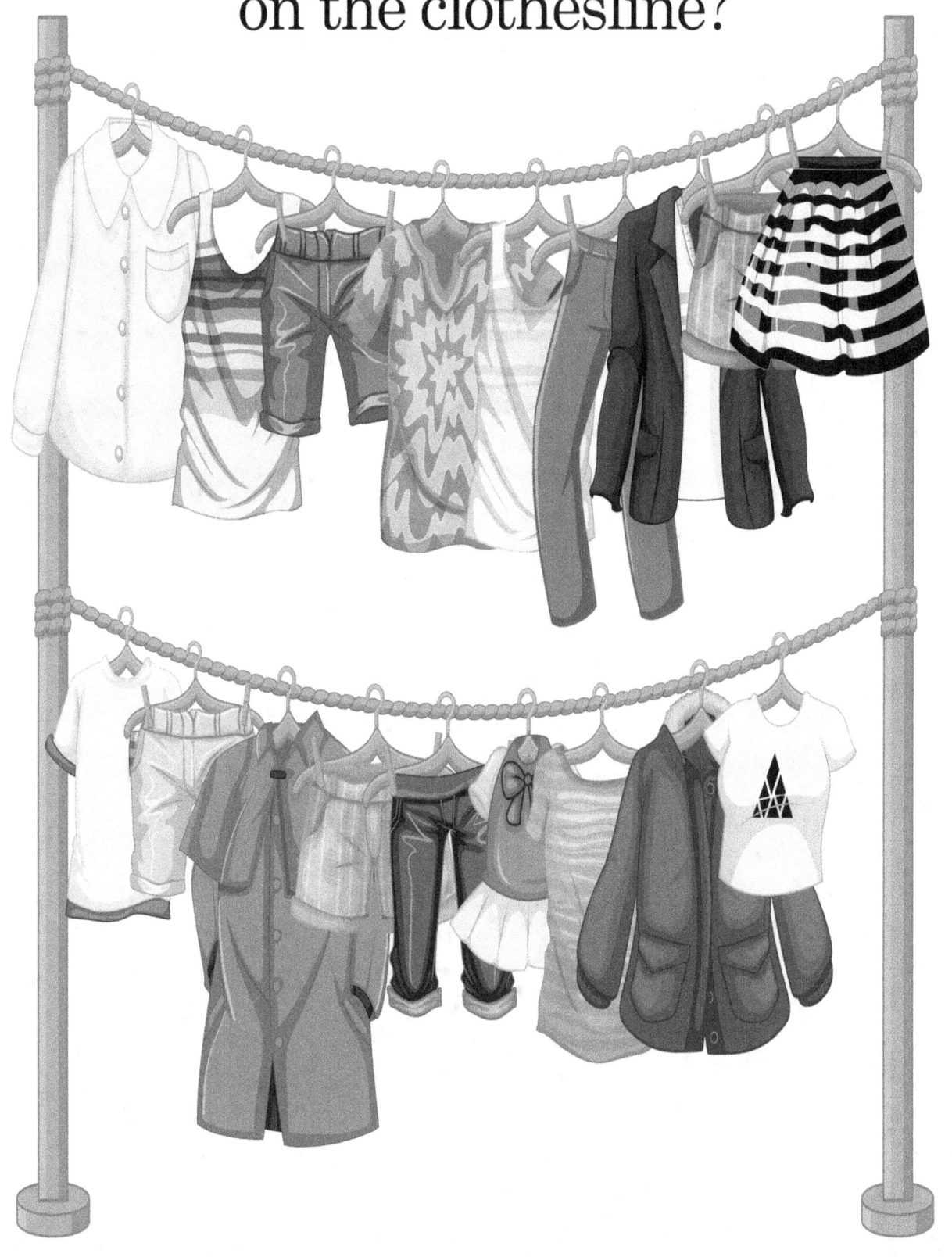

The spirit never ages. It stays forever young

Write the names of the parts of the human body

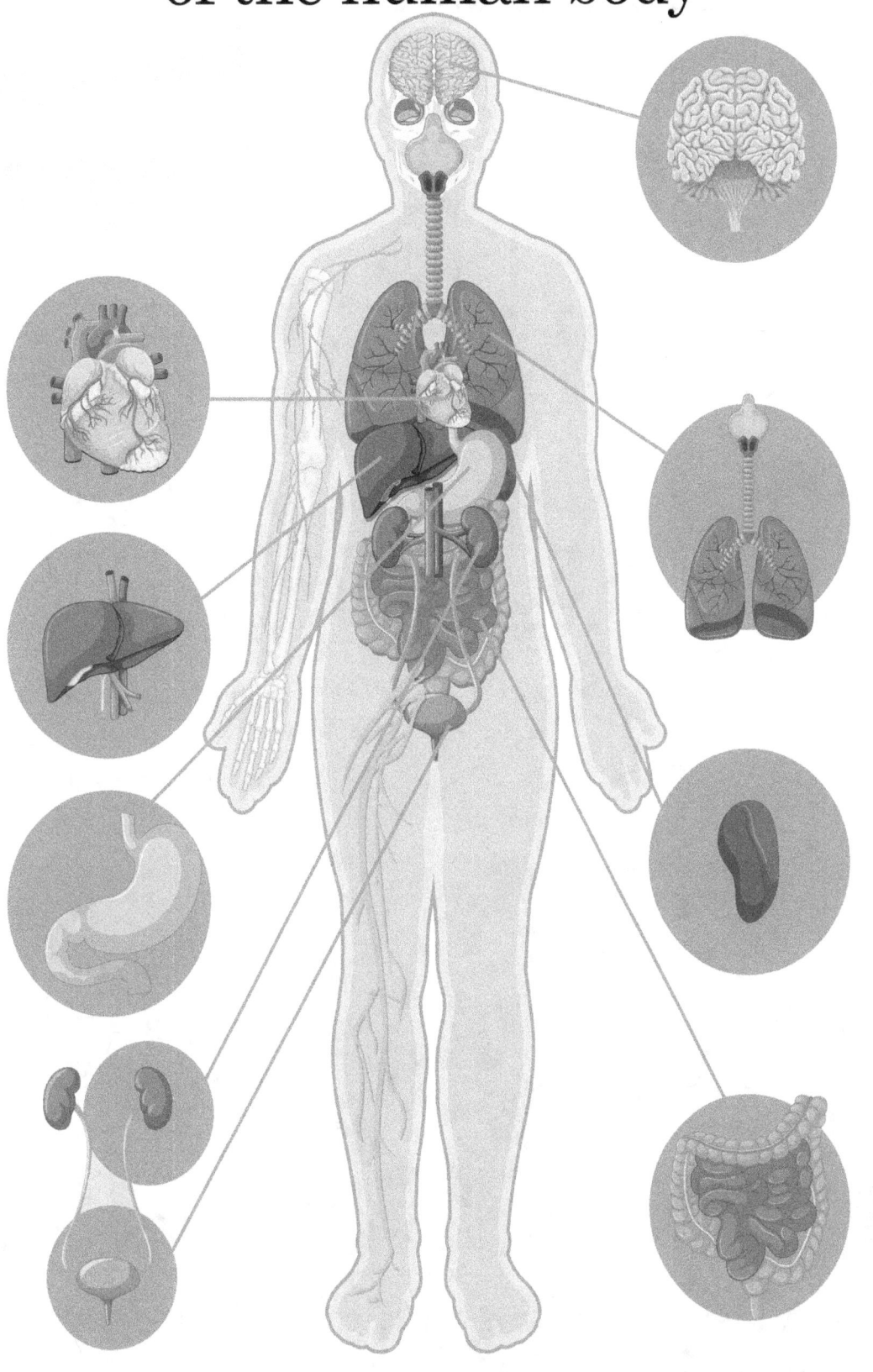

Paint each figure a different color

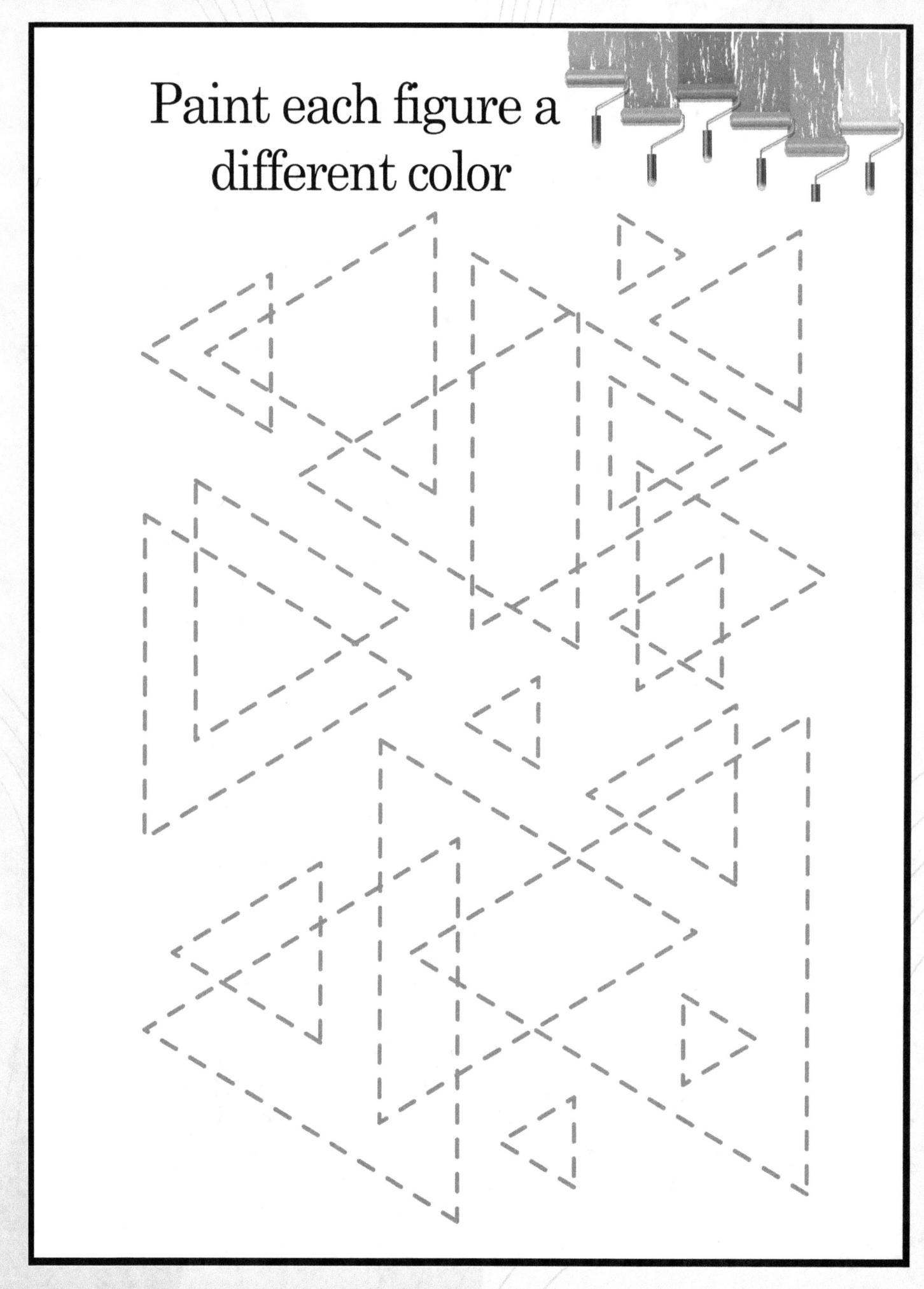

Trace

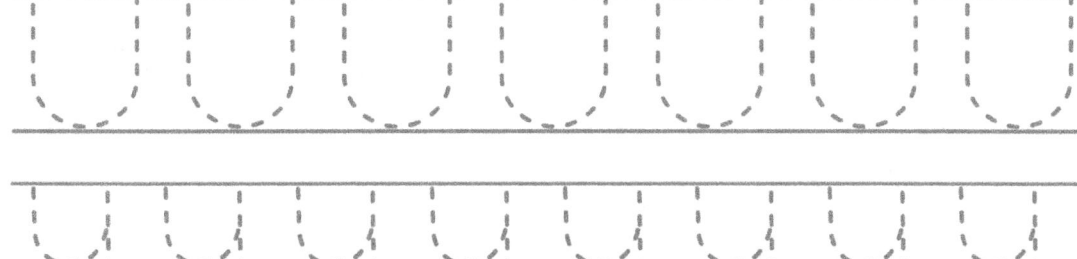

Find and color U

P Z U U M U
p
Q j W t h u i
N U T U j e v
B U L E c f u a
U U O U U P I
V U r u x m S

Connect the dots and color

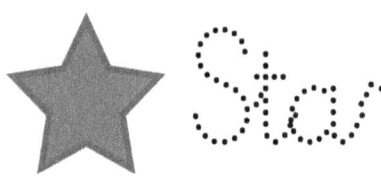 *Star* *Star* *Star*

Color *Trace*

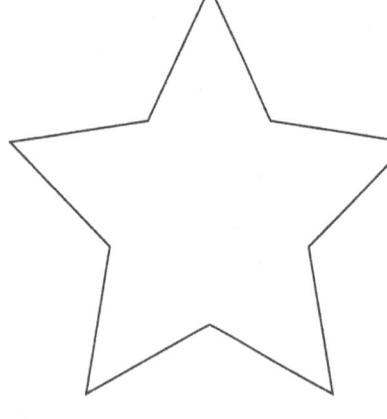

Connect the dots *Draw*

Subtraction

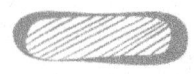

837 - 381	948 - 261	691 - 247	515 - 70
947 - 272	993 - 315	620 - 487	682 - 38
674 - 419	580 - 126	803 - 168	530 - 286
793 - 135	980 - 346	814 - 377	952 - 406

Find the exit

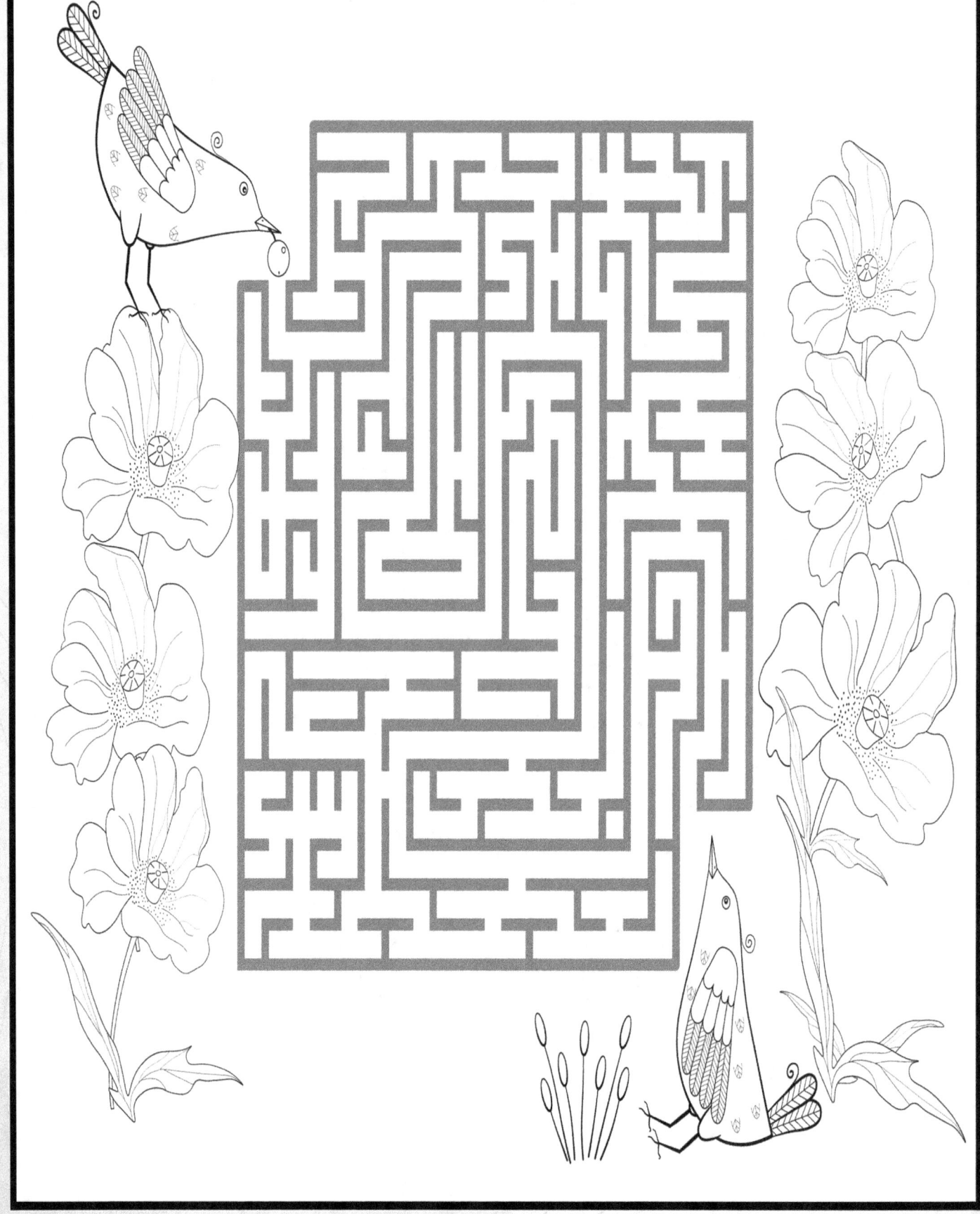

Paint each circle a different color

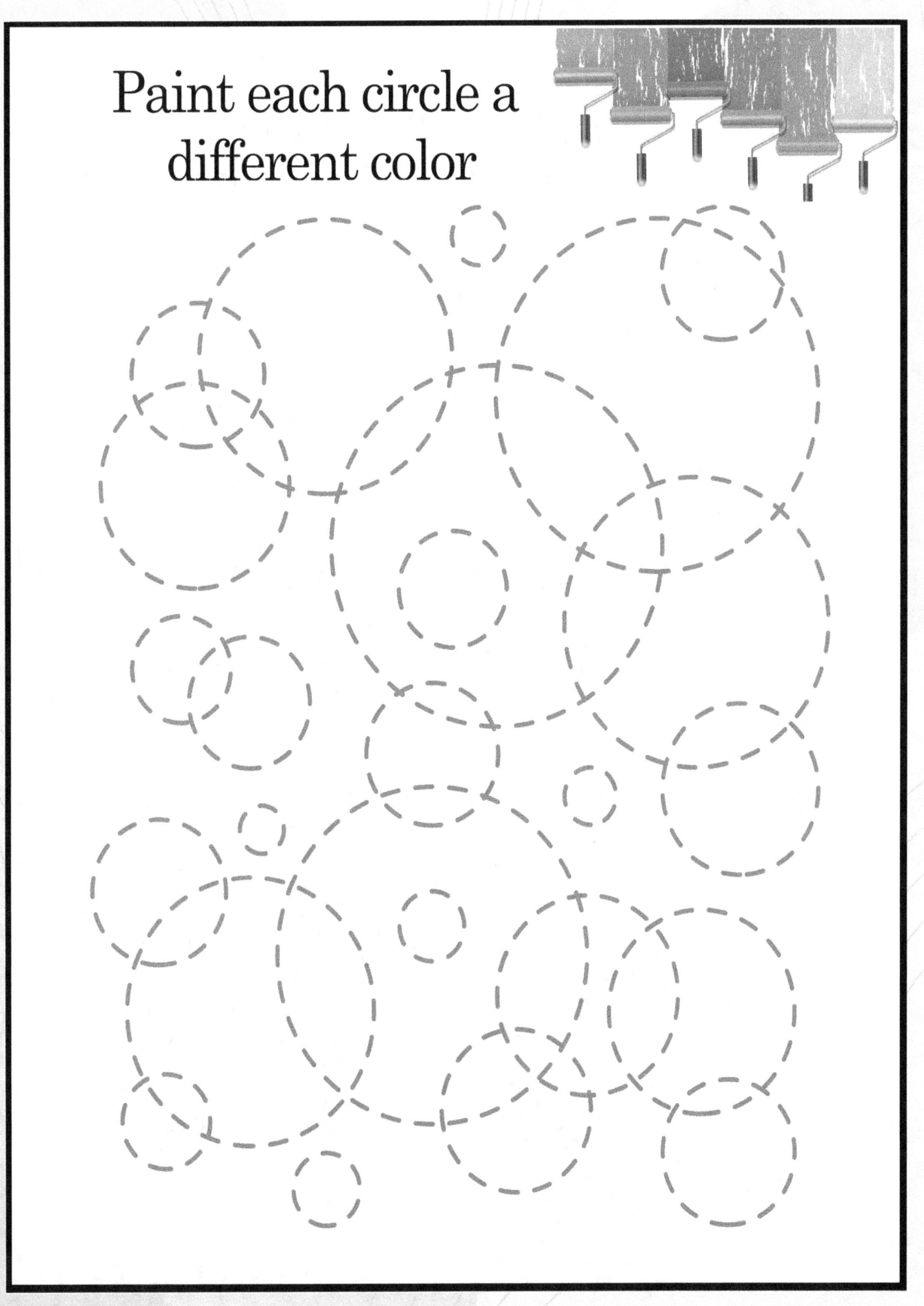

Paint by numbers

1 - Orange 2 - Blue 3 - Green 4 - Black 5 - Yellow

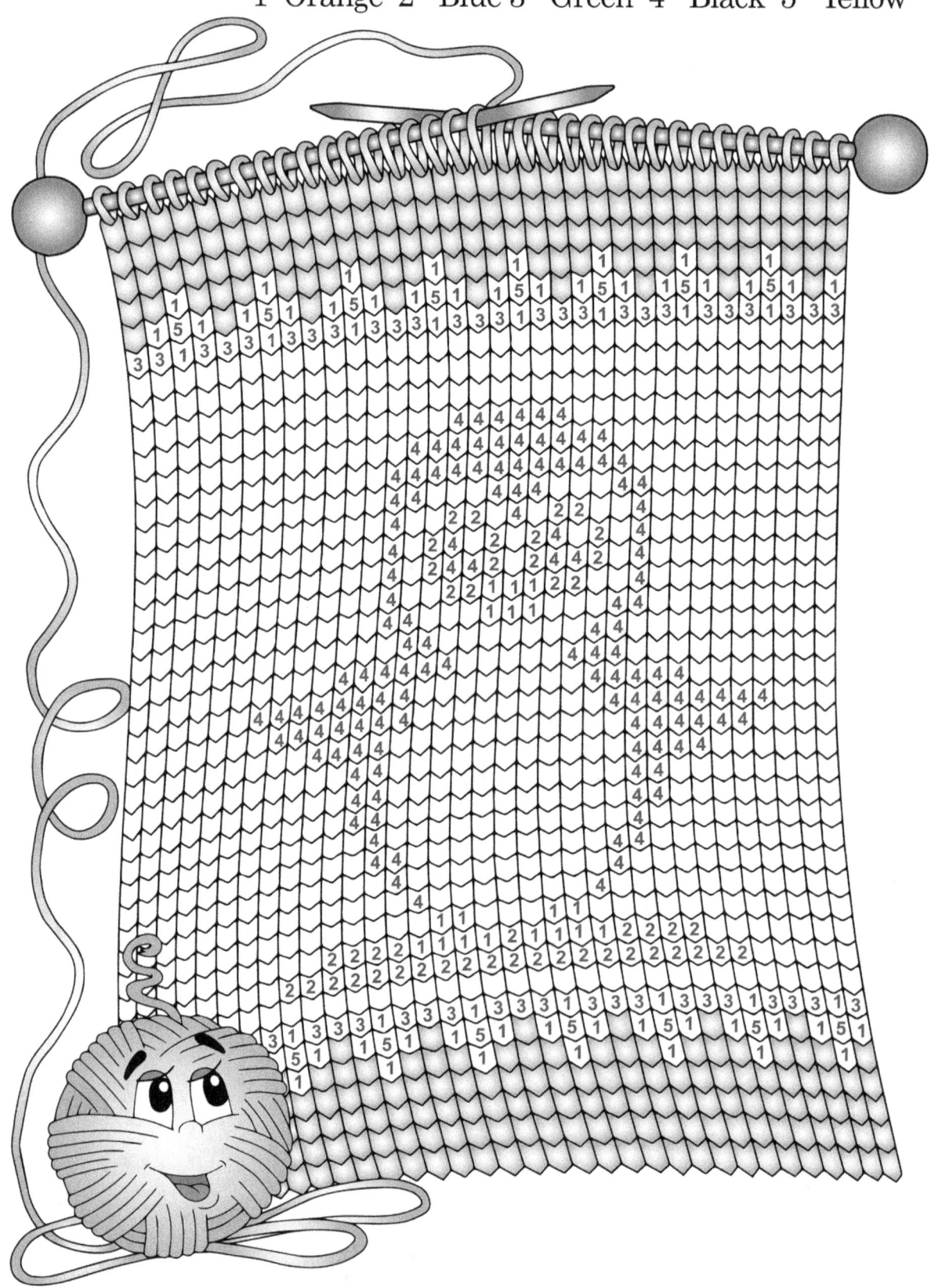

Trace the shapes

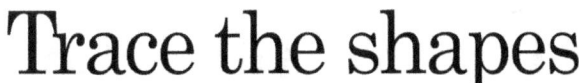

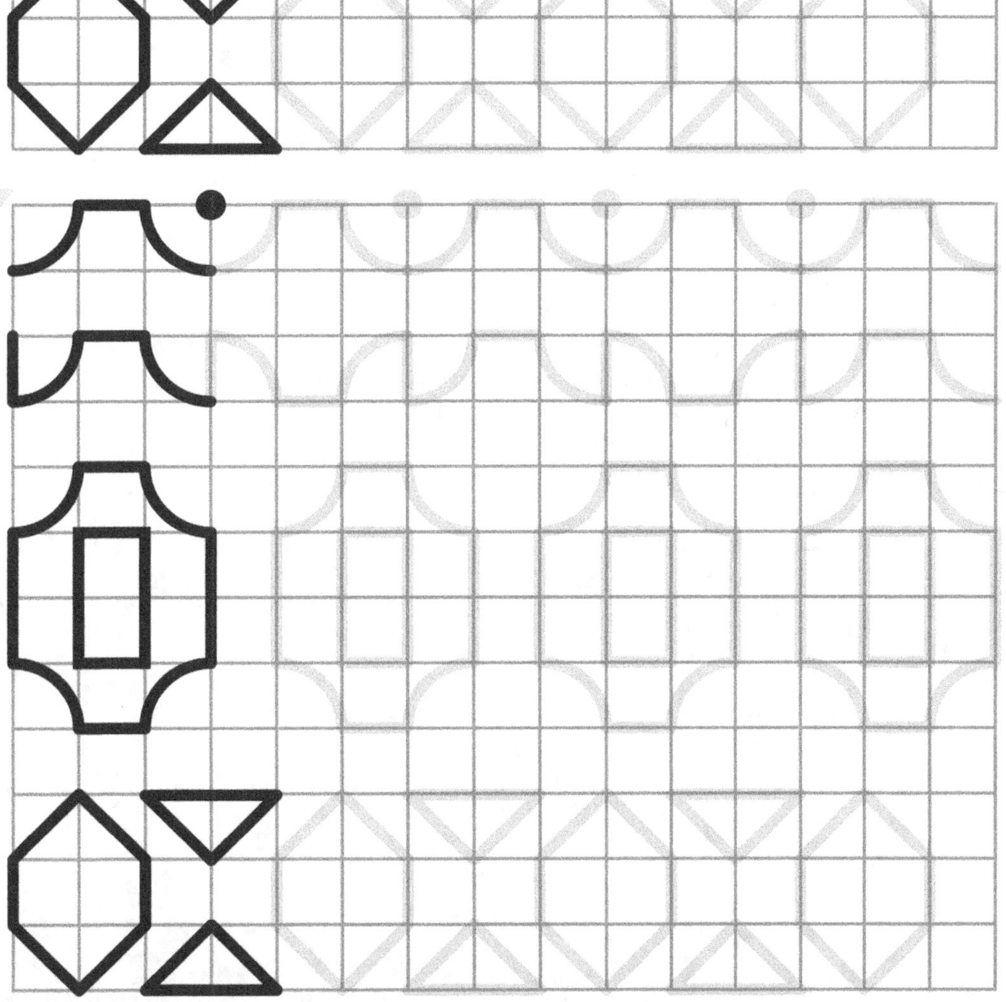

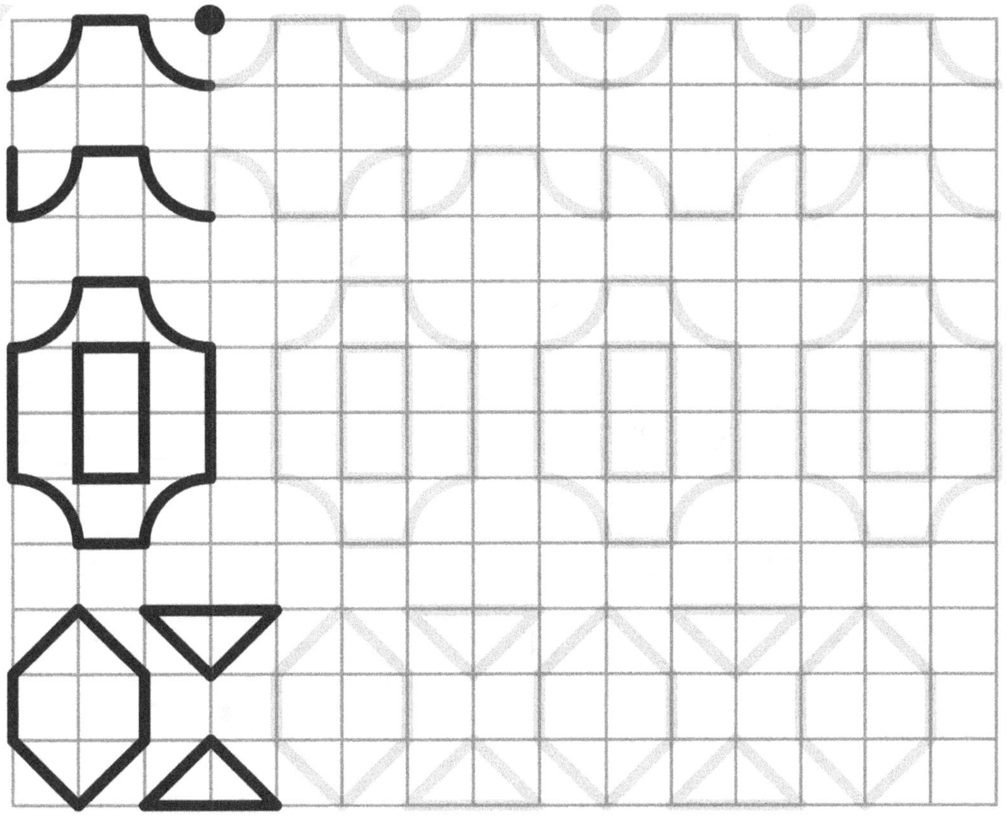

Draw and color

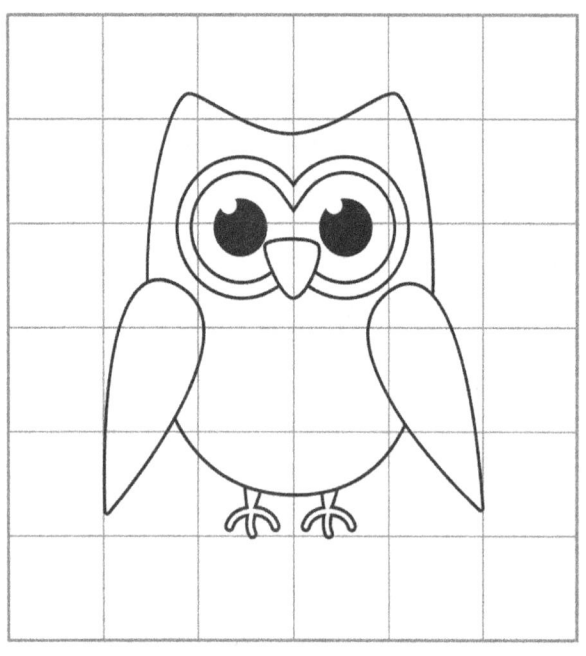

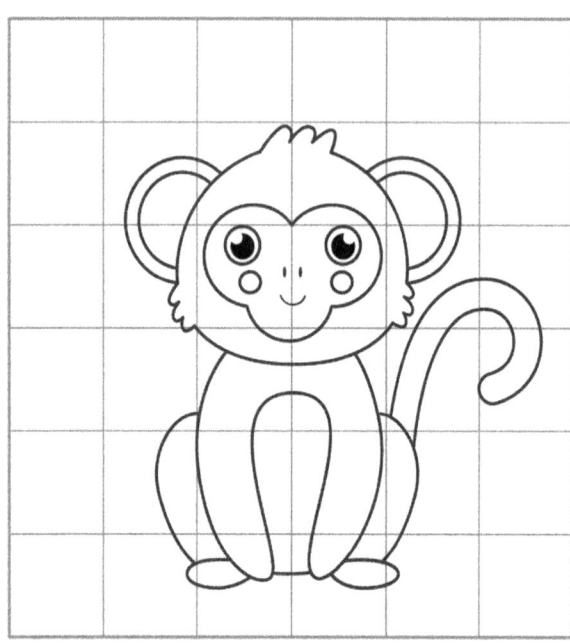

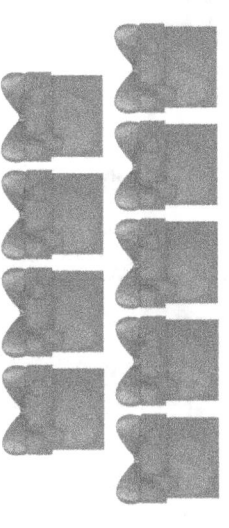

TRACE THE NUMBER

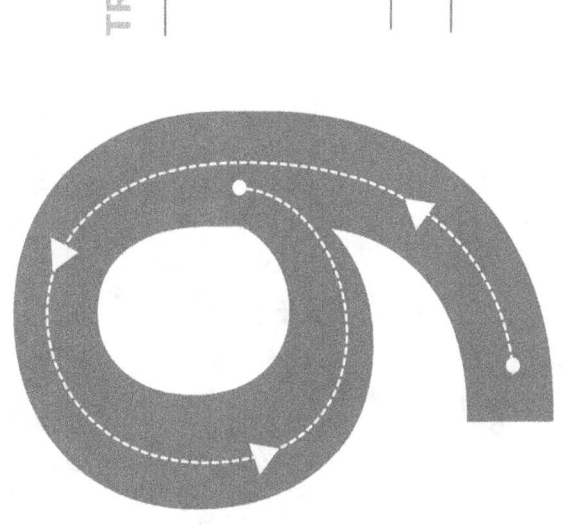

CIRCLE ALL THE NUMBER NINE

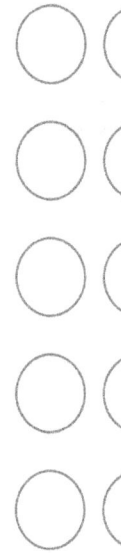
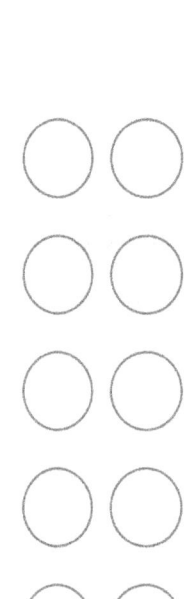

9 8 9 8 7 9
1 5 3 1 8 1
4 2 8 9 9 8
7 7

CLOLOR NINE CIRCLES

NINE

What are your great memories with your family?

_____

_____

_____

_____

_____

_____

_____

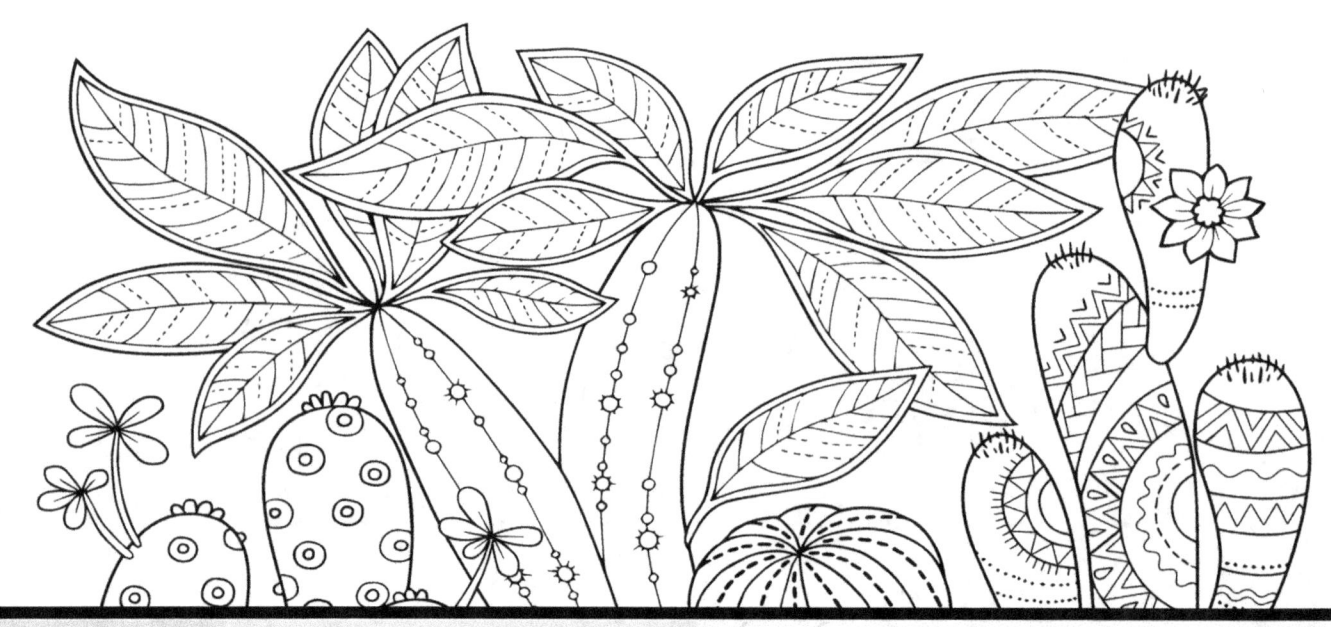

How many of each type are there?

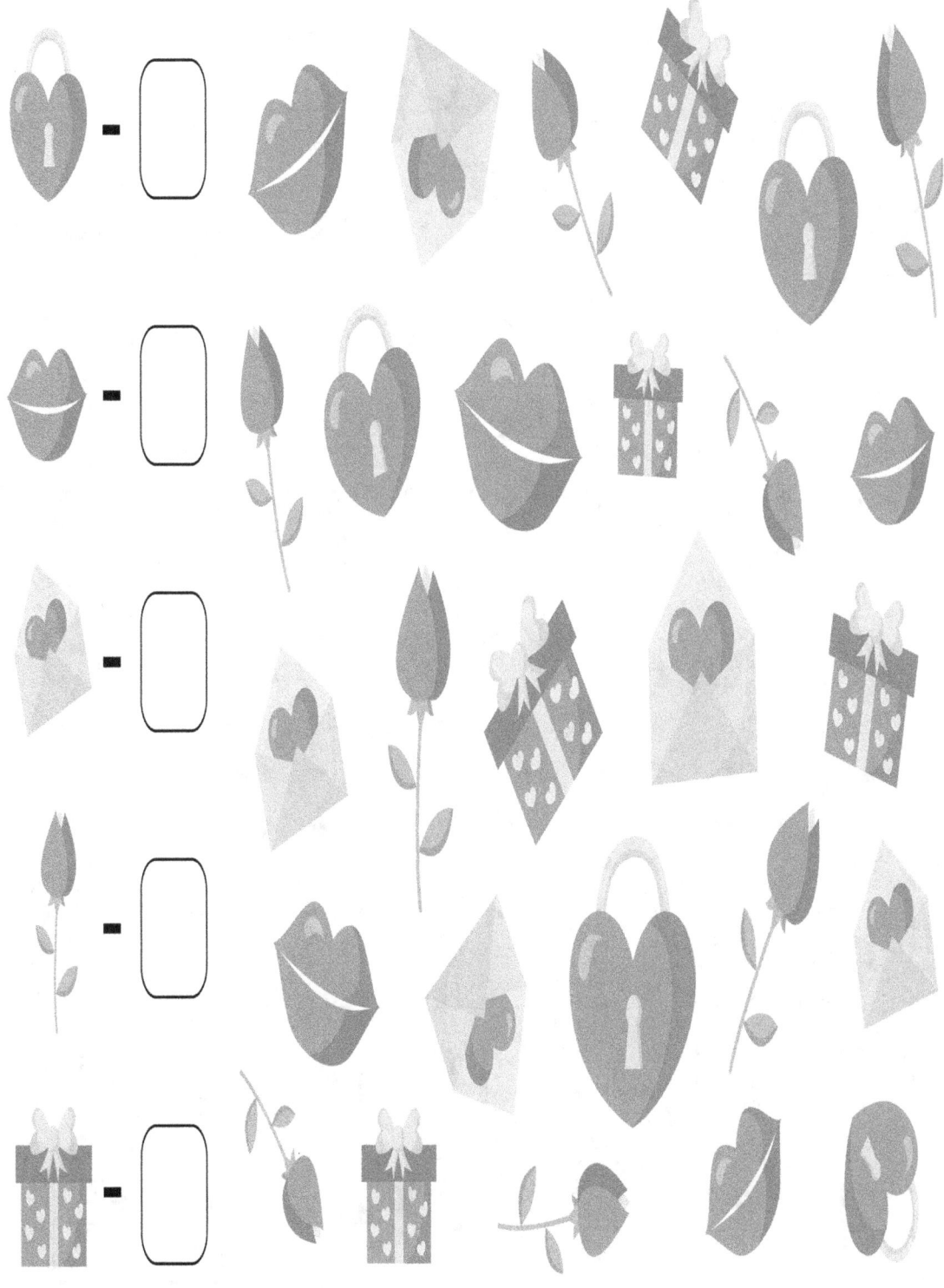

Get to number 16 going through the numbers in order

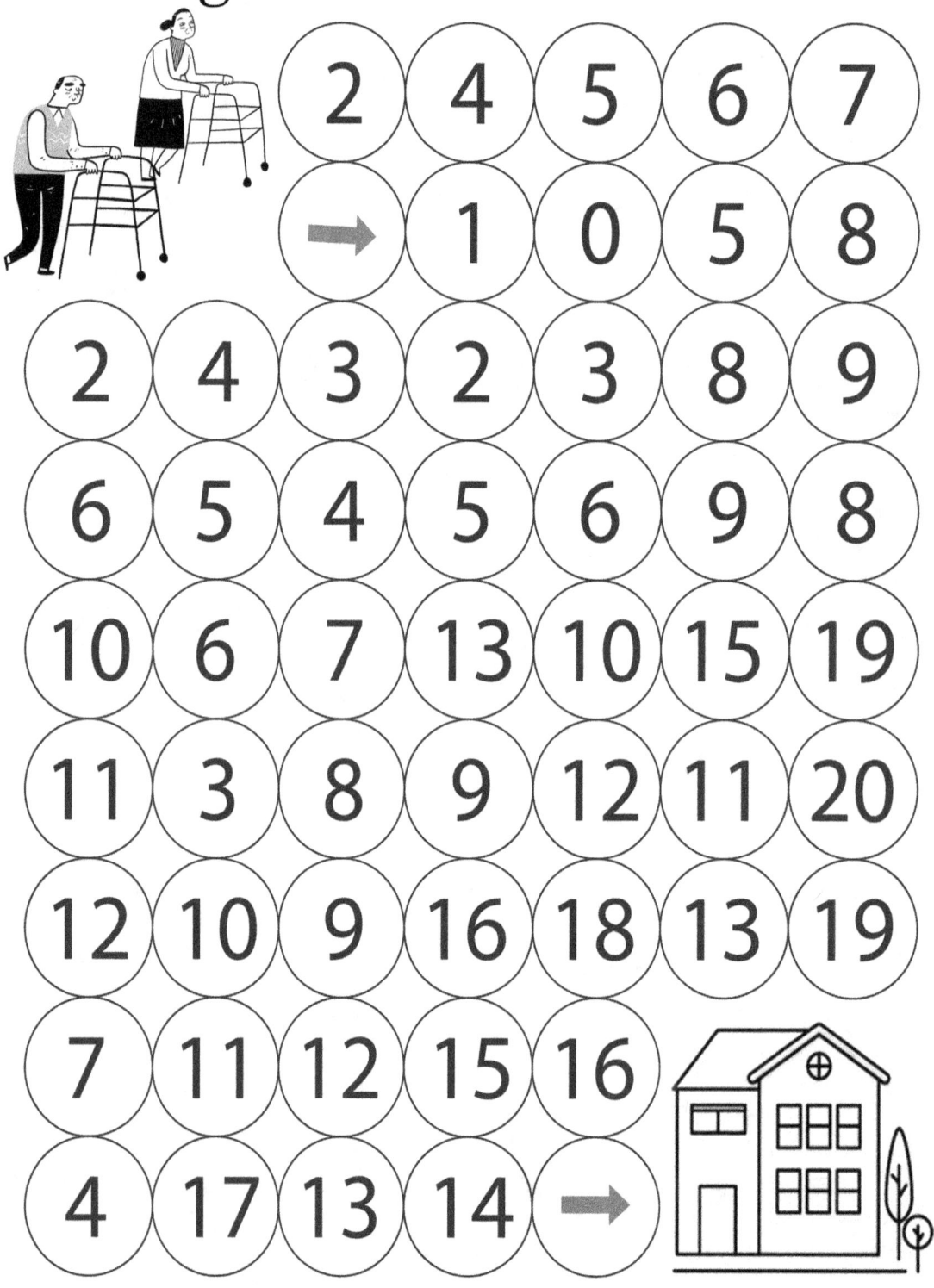

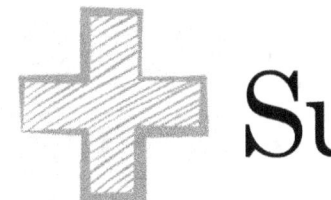 # Sums

$+\ \begin{matrix} 28 \\ 26 \end{matrix}$ $+\ \begin{matrix} 15 \\ 37 \end{matrix}$ $+\ \begin{matrix} 29 \\ 29 \end{matrix}$ $+\ \begin{matrix} 05 \\ 36 \end{matrix}$ $+\ \begin{matrix} 73 \\ 51 \end{matrix}$ $+\ \begin{matrix} 83 \\ 91 \end{matrix}$

$+\ \begin{matrix} 06 \\ 28 \end{matrix}$ $+\ \begin{matrix} 54 \\ 74 \end{matrix}$ $+\ \begin{matrix} 92 \\ 71 \end{matrix}$ $+\ \begin{matrix} 71 \\ 90 \end{matrix}$ $+\ \begin{matrix} 51 \\ 74 \end{matrix}$ $+\ \begin{matrix} 08 \\ 38 \end{matrix}$

$+\ \begin{matrix} 39 \\ 28 \end{matrix}$ $+\ \begin{matrix} 28 \\ 39 \end{matrix}$ $+\ \begin{matrix} 60 \\ 82 \end{matrix}$ $+\ \begin{matrix} 90 \\ 71 \end{matrix}$ $+\ \begin{matrix} 71 \\ 62 \end{matrix}$ $+\ \begin{matrix} 72 \\ 73 \end{matrix}$

$+\ \begin{matrix} 29 \\ 06 \end{matrix}$ $+\ \begin{matrix} 28 \\ 45 \end{matrix}$ $+\ \begin{matrix} 54 \\ 71 \end{matrix}$ $+\ \begin{matrix} 17 \\ 19 \end{matrix}$ $+\ \begin{matrix} 64 \\ 63 \end{matrix}$ $+\ \begin{matrix} 73 \\ 63 \end{matrix}$

When you were a kid, what made you happy the most?

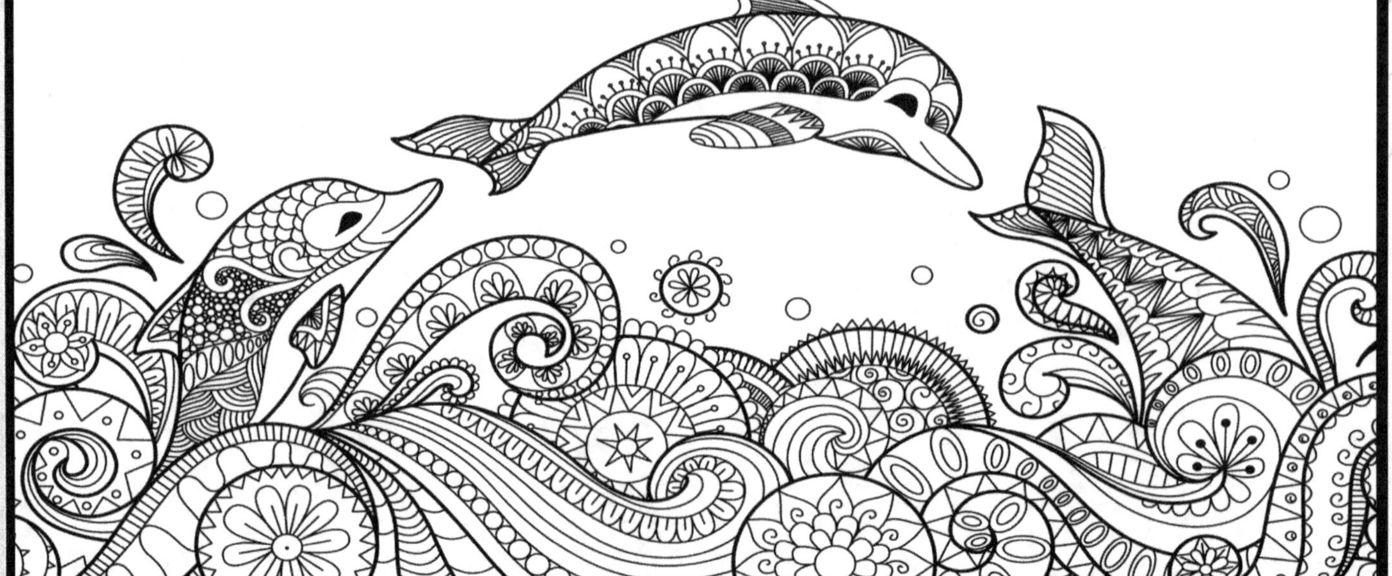

_____

_____

_____

_____

_____

_____

_____

How many figures are there of each type?

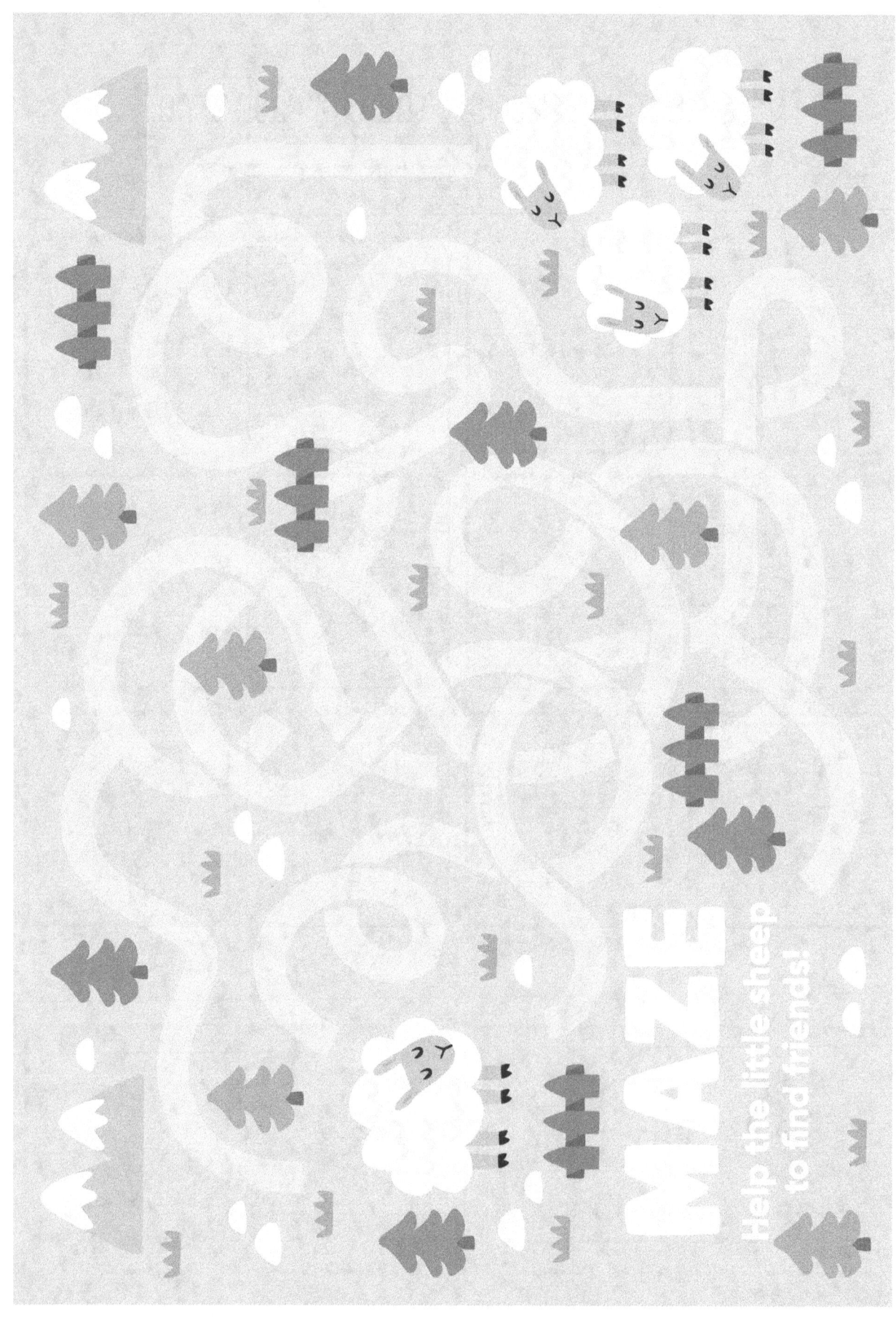

MAZE

Help the little sheep
to find friends!

Find the 7 differences

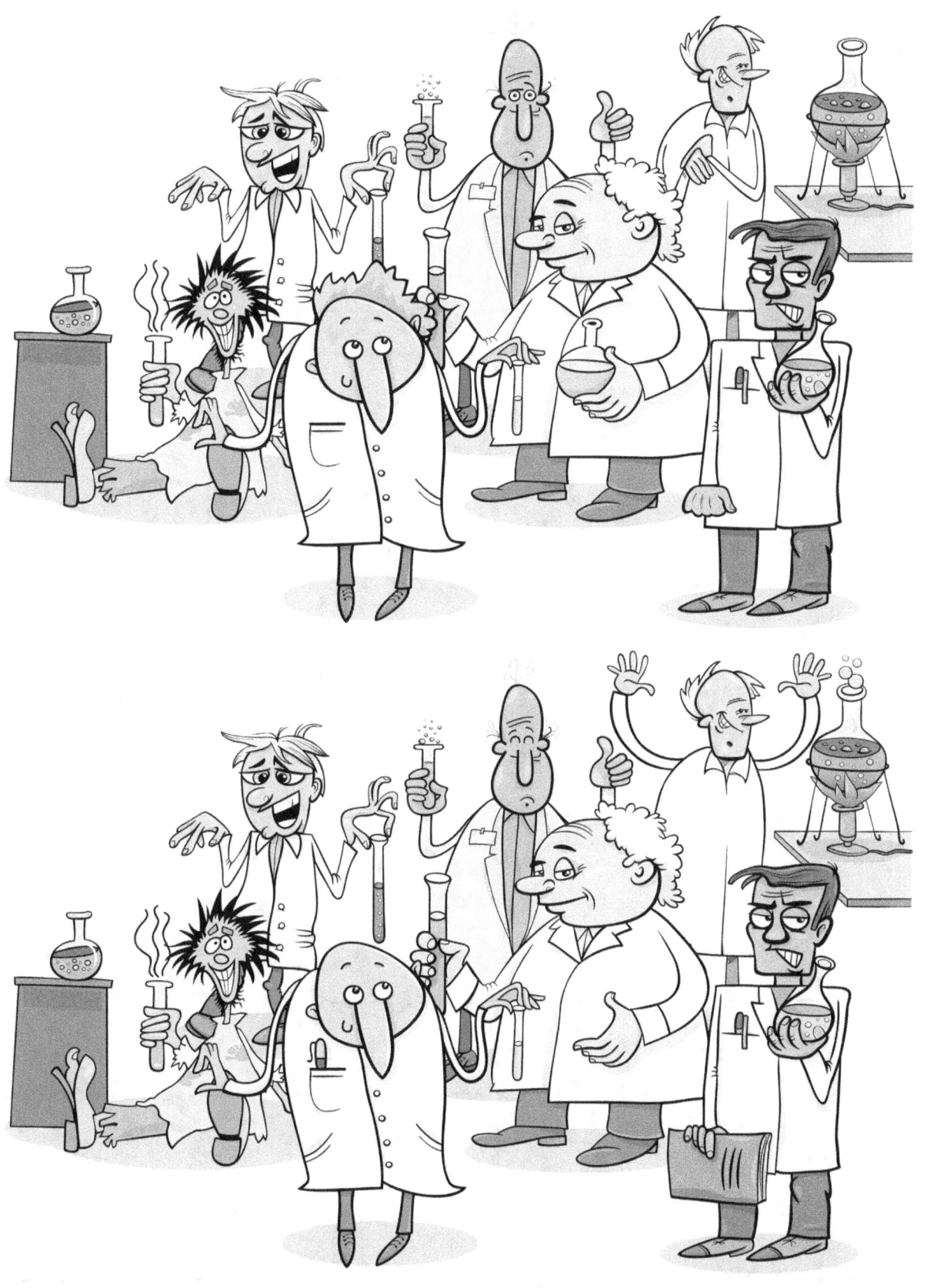

Find the exit

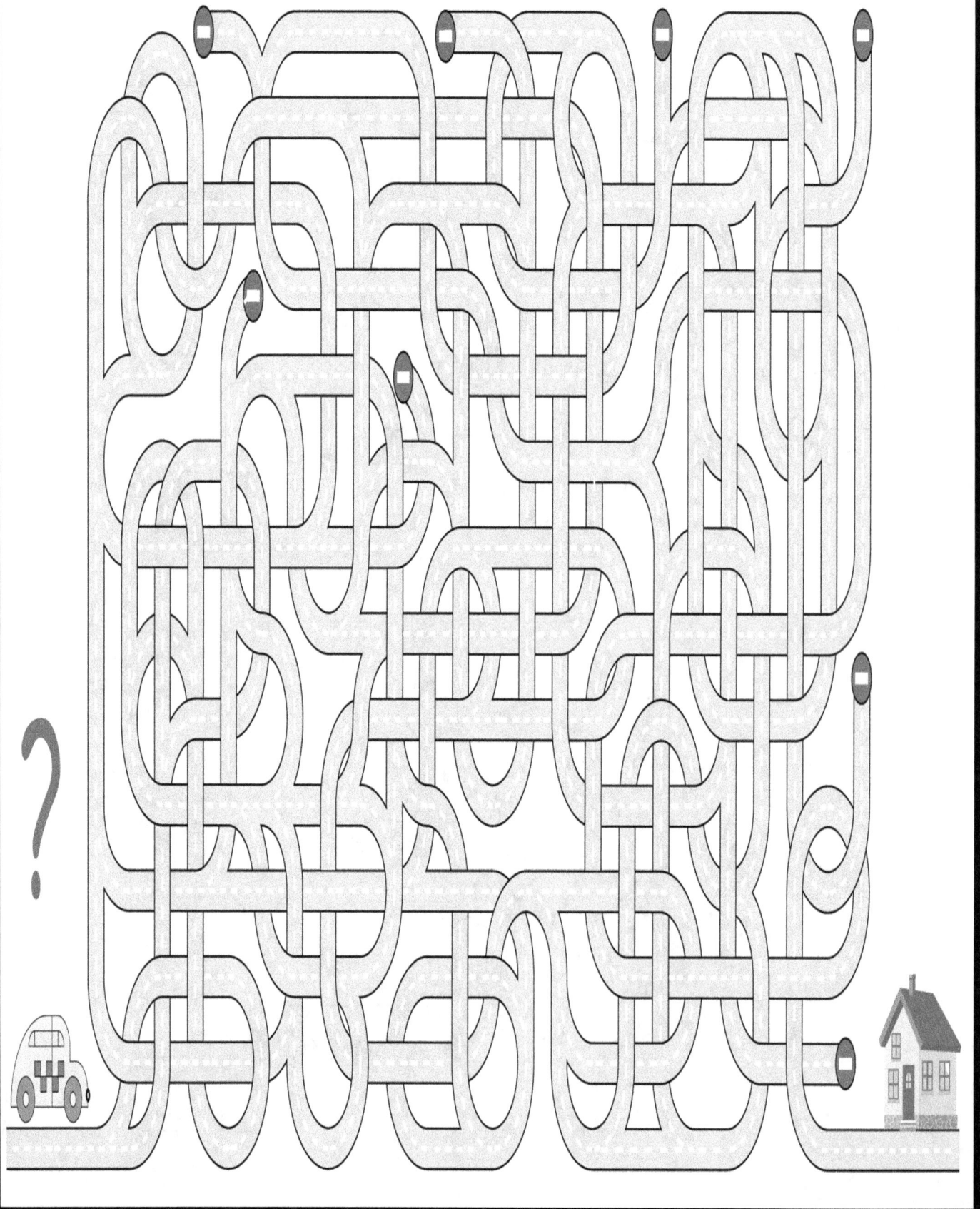

Find the identical pair of musicians

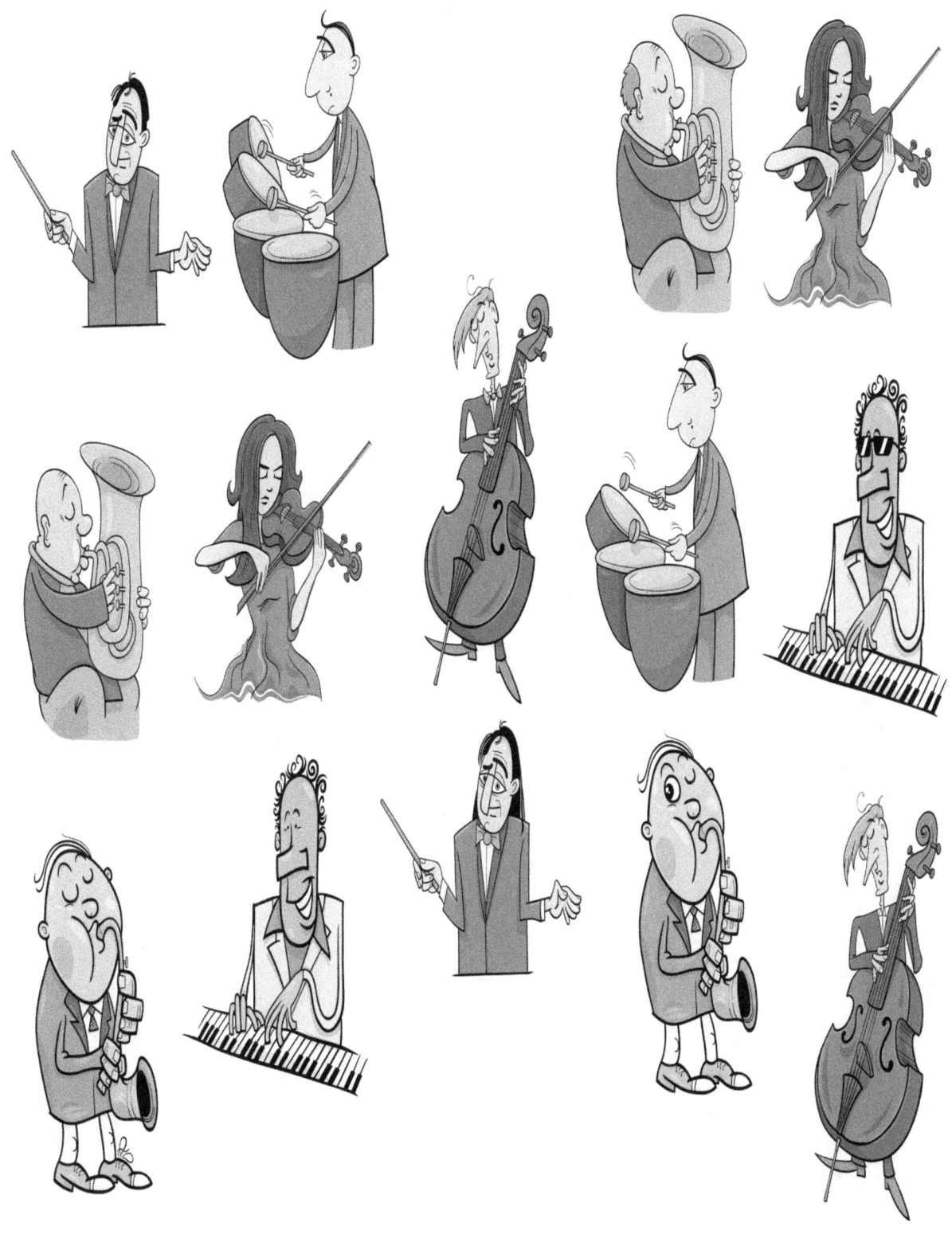

Tracing the numbers

1 1 1 1 1 1 1 1 1 1

2 2 2 2 2 2 2 2 2 2

3 3 3 3 3 3 3 3 3 3

4 4 4 4 4 4 4 4 4 4

5 5 5 5 5 5 5 5 5 5

6 6 6 6 6 6 6 6 6 6

7 7 7 7 7 7 7 7 7 7

8 8 8 8 8 8 8 8 8 8

9 9 9 9 9 9 9 9 9 9

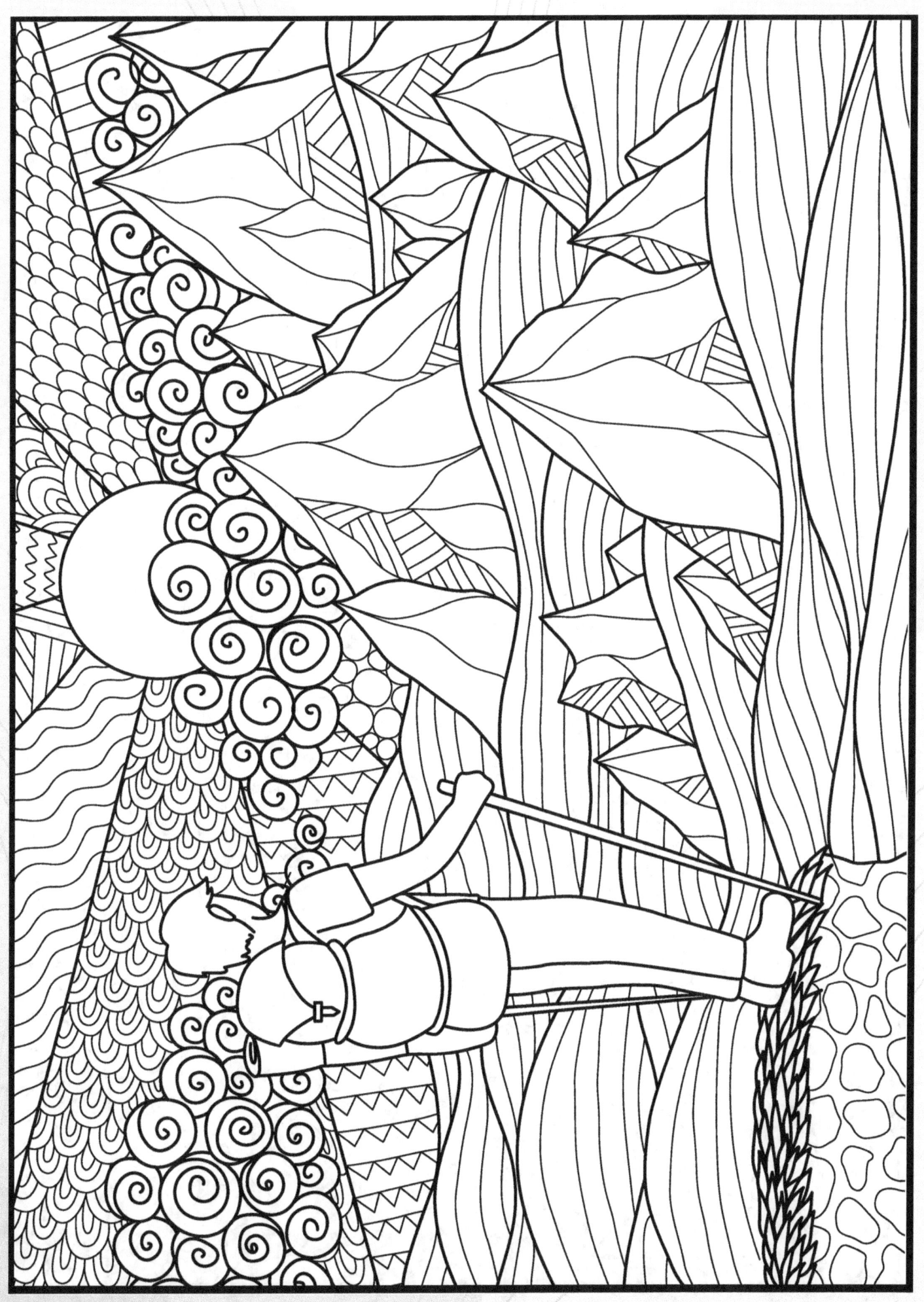

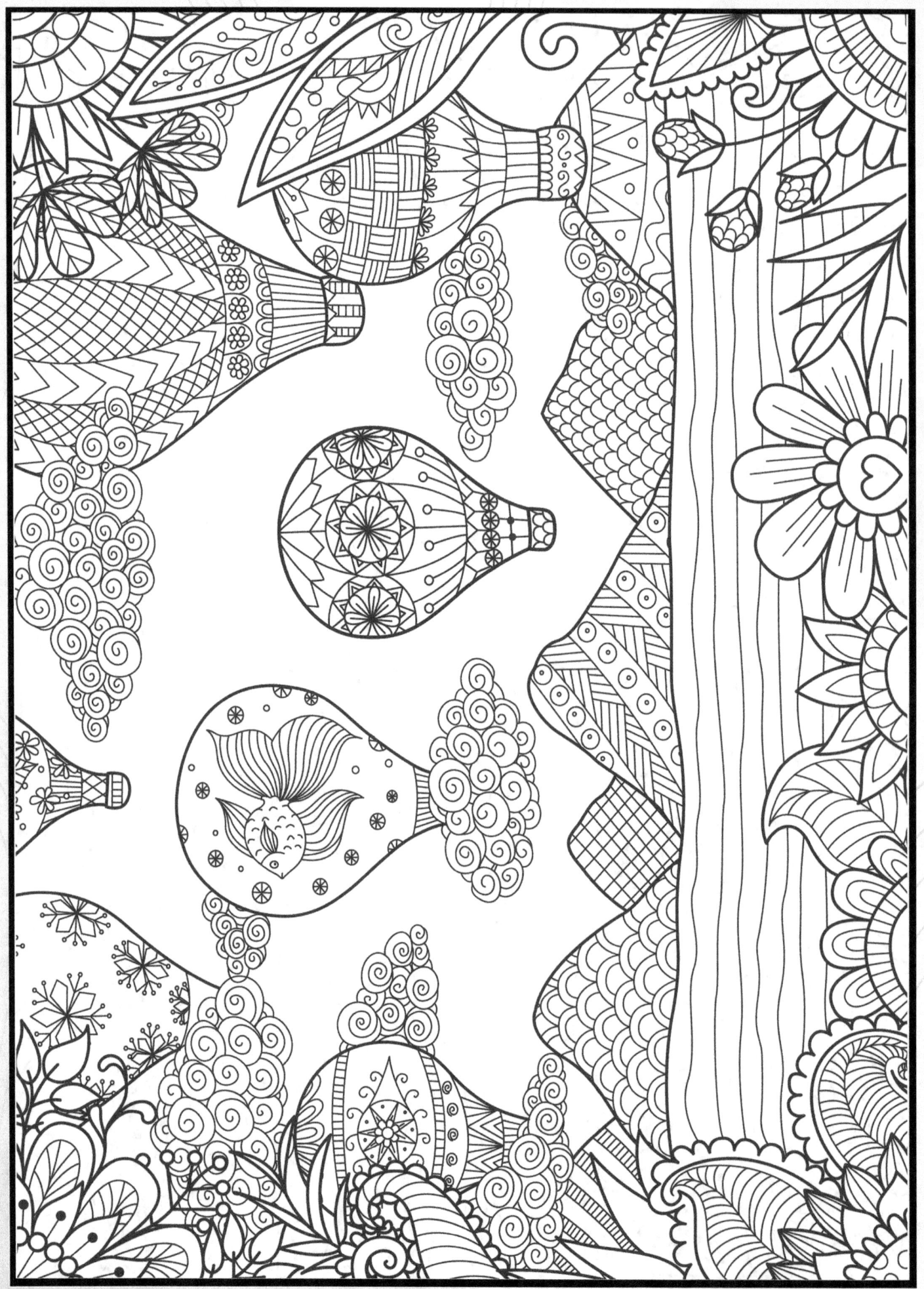

We sincerely hope that your loved ones had an

entertaining and enjoyable time.

It is a real pleasure for us to design books for people

so important in our lives.

We would love to see their creations in the comments...

Alber Doncos

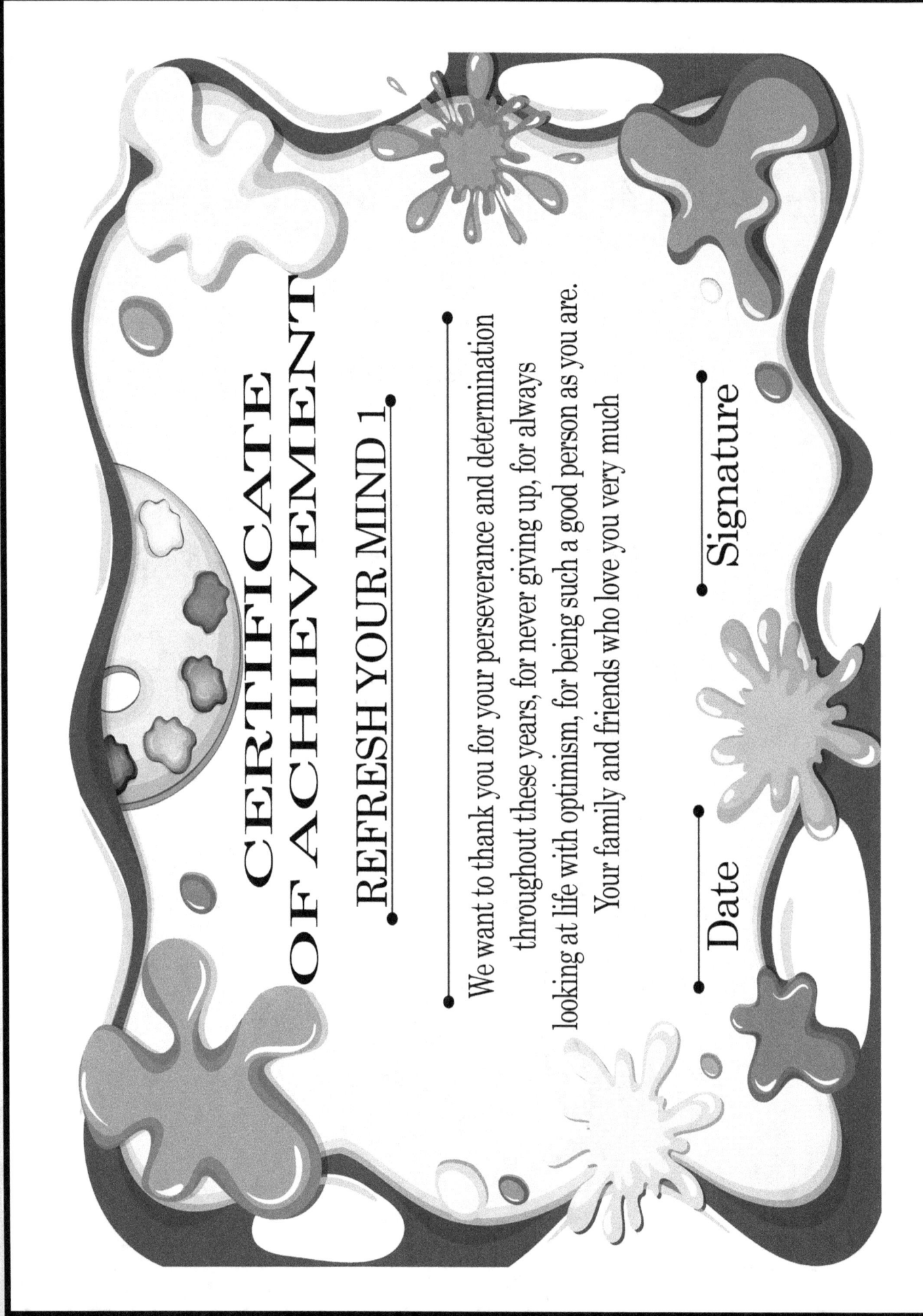

CERTIFICATE
OF ACHIEVEMENT

REFRESH YOUR MIND 1

We want to thank you for your perseverance and determination throughout these years, for never giving up, for always looking at life with optimism, for being such a good person as you are.
Your family and friends who love you very much

Signature

Date

www.ingramcontent.com/pod-product-compliance
Lightning Source LLC
Chambersburg PA
CBHW082147230526
45467CB00043B/2398